PIONEERS COMPANION WORKBOOK:

Acupuncture Treatment Plans and Pathways

AMBER ROSE

Library of Congress Cataloging-in-Publication Data

Rose, Amber

1. Holistic Medicine   2. Bee Venom Therapy   3. Acupuncture

I. Title   615.89 RO

Desktop Publishing by Forever Amber Publishing

Illustrations by Shonne N. Farrell, B.F.A.

Foreword by Dr. Barry Fruchter

Introduction by Tom Ingegno, MSOM. L.Ac.

Copyright @ 2015 1st Edition

Published in the United States by Forever Amber Publishing.

Grateful acknowledgement is made to the following for permission to reprint previously published material:

Bee in Balance: A Guide to Healing the Whole Person with Honeybees, Oriental Medicine, & Common Sense;

Excerpt from Dianne Connelly, All Sickness is Homesickness. Columbia, MD: The Traditional Acupuncture Institute, 1993, reprinted with permission.

Library of Congress Catalog Card Number:

ISBN -13: 978-1517178222

ISBN -10: 1517178223

Library of Congress Catalog Card Number: 2015914979

CreateSpace Independent Publishing Platform

North Charleston, South Carolina

DEDICATED TO DOV ROSE

AND ALL MY PIONEERS

TABLE OF CONTENTS

ACKNOWLEDGMENTS

ON A PERSONAL NOTE:

- Reuben Skye Rose-Redwood, my son—who kept me going all these years . . . who believed in me, who had many dinners alone because I was working late. . . and when we ate together we often had bees, tweezers, spray bottles on the table.

- My wonderful husband-cousin, Dov (who has loved me all his life)…my beloved companion, who encouraged me every step of the way. He always made sure I ate and brought me all my meals while I was busy typing, who cleaned the house and walked the dog, and waited on me hand and foot, after a long day at work himself. . . Dov, I could not have written this book without your loving support and TLC.

- To my devoted friends, Tatiana Love, Wendie Kidwell, Deborah Einbender, Jonathan Klate, Matty Young, Meg Mills, Natasha Rabin, Shonagh Home, Buffi Young, Cheryl Thiruvathukal, Nancy Lacantore Rauhofer, Grace Madden, Shirley McClurg, Lorena Gonzelez, Azalea Lemoine, Deb Elder, Shalini Kruger, Kari Krug, Nancy Rigg, Jean Durscher, Jodie Drury-Roznos, Belinda Tveit Williams, Patty Preston, Jennifer Lanett, Mindy Boyett, Andy Turner,Grace Madden, Leo Montgomery, and Hubert Duke, …Thank you all for your constant emotional love and support over all these years.

- To my sister Nomi Rosen, her husband Ralph, her daughter Kate and son - in - law Pat... Thank you for welcoming me with open arms. I love you all.

- To my wonderful sister - in - law, Kathi Thomas Rosen… who is my inspiration….I love you to the moon and back. To my niece, Amanda who loves animals and her future husband Brad, plus my musical nephew Josh….And someone who will always have a special place in my heart, my brother Seth Michael Rosen. We all love and miss you.

- To my mother and father, Lillian and Sidney Rosen, who I miss very dearly and who in their own quiet way were always "rootin' for me."

- For all my 12-step friends, especially the women in the Tuesday morning meeting, who gave me the courage to go on with my life when I felt discouraged . . .

THANKS TO NOTEWORTHY "BEE PEOPLE":

- Charlie Mraz, King of Bee Venom Therapy, my first mentor and true friend and his children.

- Pat Wagner, my first teacher.

- Cheryl Thiruvathukal, who truly believes in me and encouraged my work with bees.

- Nancy Lacontore Rauhofer for her encouragement and suggestions.

- Buffi Young for her help in creating a wonderful, supportive FB community, Pioneers: Healing Lyme with Bee Venom Therapy. It is a sanctuary of hope for me to share my knowledge. And special thanks to Buffi and her daughter Sophie for their technical wizardry.

- Deb Elder's enthusiastic belief in Bee Venom Therapy. Thanks for creating so many Apitherapy pages and radio blogshows.

- Special thanks to all the patients and loved ones on all the BVT Lyme pages, without whose generous sharings I could not have created this book.

- Sandy Berg Liccardi, Shonagh Home, Angela Hartnett, and Tigerlily who have helped me create some workshops and artwork.

- All of my Pioneers on FB

- And Charlie Koenen for encouraging me to reprint my book, Bee in Balance…without which I would not have access to the drawings for this workbook.

- Tom Ingegno, Jennifer Brown, Jennifer Lannett and others for wanting to study with me.

- And for Dr. Ahmed Hegazi who invited me to speak at the Immunology Summit in Texas, September, 2015. And who appointed me to the editorial board of the new peer-reviewed "International Journal of Apitherapy."

- Thanks to all the patients who let me sting them with bees in acupuncture points. . . for practicing "living acupuncture" on them

- To all the groups that invited me to speak.

- Special thanks to Charlie Mraz who made me feel special and believed in my ideas about combining acupuncture and bee venom therapy . . . who gave me three of his best hives . . . who initiated me into the world of bees on a 13 hour drive from Vermont to Maryland with those hives in the back of the station wagon. The hives opened up and the bees were crawling all over us for hours and neither of us got stung . . . .and who showed me everything he knew about bee venom collection. And special thanks to his daughters Michelle and Marna for all their support.

FOR THOSE WHO HELPED DIRECTLY WITH THE BOOK

- Shonne N. Farrell, M.B.A., created the illustrations.

- My son Reuben Rose-Redwood who helped me make sure my margins and pagination were correct.

- Tom Ingegno & Barry Fruchter for introductory material.

AND REGARDING ACUPUNCTURE

- Jonathan, Reuben, and Charlotte Klate who inspired me to go to acupuncture school.

- The staff at Traditional Acupuncture Institute.

- Dr. Rind for believing in me and sending me patients.

- All my acupuncture patients who taught me more than I could learn from any book.

- To all my acupuncture/massage students who always remind me just how much I love teaching.

- All my special friends, students and colleagues at NY College of Health Professions, The Swedish Institute, and East-West College for their love and encouragement. Thank you for knowing and understanding who I really am and what I came here to do on this earth.

AND MOST OF ALL

- Those wonderful honeybees who gave their lives so selflessly to help us heal ourselves. The honeybees are the only creatures on the earth that improve the environment and do not prey on any other species. We have a lot to learn from them.

FOREWORD

THE LADY AND THE MIRACLE

I first read Amber Rose's magnum opus, **Bee in Balance**, in 2005. From the first page on, it grabbed me and would not let me go. Amber is masterful at interweaving personal narrative, testimony, history, western biology, and Asian medicine into a seamless web and then applying it to cover and enclose all our individual stories. As she says, she has been a healer all her life. Her own healing journey – from educator and psychotherapist to acupuncturist to apitherapist – is so vast and sweeping that it gives us all the feeling that she is telling us our own story, reflecting back to us our own experience, strength, and hope, and permitting us to move forward in our lives. Her subtitle ends with the words "and common sense," which seem to prophesy her latest book, *Pioneers: Healing Lyme with Bee Venom Therapy*.

Amber Rose is certainly a caring practitioner of Bee Venom Therapy, BVT, specifically for Lyme patients. She is very likely a saint. Even without reading her books, all that's needed is talking to anyone who has been on a phone consult with her, asked her a question on her FaceBook group, Pioneers: Healing Lyme with Bee Venom Therapy, or attended one of her BVT workshops and possibly gotten stung and cared for by her. I was lucky enough to attend several such workshops in various parts of the USA. She is also well-known in Canada and Mexico and, via FaceBook, in Britain and many other countries. The key element of Amber's practice is love.

Amber often tells the story of her first acquaintance with the use of honeybees to treat autoimmune diseases and infections. After nearly ten years of treating clients with Five Element Acupuncture, the ancient kind that takes the emotions as well as the physical body symptoms into account, her discovery of BVT quickly led her to the idea of combining beestings with acupuncture, of stinging in acupuncture points for greater effectiveness against Lyme and related infections. As she says, she thought she invented the idea...until she visited China, a few months later, accompanied by others including Charles Mraz, the famed "King of Bee Venom Therapy," and discovered that the Chinese had been practicing bee-acupuncture for 3, 000 years! All this is to say that not only is Amber an original thinker and a quick study but also a woman deeply imbued with humility. She never ever charges for BVT and she has deliberately lowered the cost of Pioneers so as to do the greatest good for the greatest number of patients. She gives so freely of her time and energy that she is often still awake at 2 AM, her time, helping clients on Mountain or Pacific Time – via telephone or FaceBook-- deal with medical crises. Once she spent most of Christmas dinner with her family in another room on the phone with someone whose patient had gone into anaphylactic shock, counseling the practitioner until the patient was out of danger. Then, with an apology, she rejoined her family for Christmas dinner! Amber never attributes her ability to heal to herself, only to the "sacred" bees and to the human body's ability to fight disease and heal itself.

And one more thing about Rev. Dr. Amber Rose: the depth and breadth of her learning is the equal of her humility. Her title reflects study at the New Seminary in NYC 20 years ago, her ordination as an Interfaith Minister, and her doctorate, all done in the name of healing, protecting the right to heal, and bringing people together as clients, practitioners, and friends. The same is true of her BA in Philosophical Psychology, awarded at the University of Chicago with Special Honors by her advisor, the famed humanist philosopher Dr. Hannah Arendt, of her MSW from the University of Iowa, where she was herself a "pioneer" in awarding life experience college credit to people healing themselves in rehab for drug or alcohol addiction, and of her L.Ac. degree from the Traditional Acupuncture Institute in Columbia, Maryland, where she was taught and supervised by revolutionary thinkers in the field of Oriental Medicine and by the world-renowned Dr. J. R. Worsley. Friends report that after months they had no idea whatsoever that Amber had these degrees, this certification, this experience – because she does not wave it around like a flag of self-promotion. In fact, Amber Rose is not at all about self-promotion. She's all about giving from the heart, giving of herself. Her son calls her "Mama Teresa," and indeed the comparison is a good one. The daughter of a family that cared about poor and working people and gave of itself, she has continued the tradition.

Amber Rose truly is a saint. But her new book on understanding acupuncture – specifically tailored to the needs of Lyme patients and healers – is no difficult and mystery-laden biblical text – though it may become, like her other books, a kind of "Bible" of BVT for Lyme. Instead, it is an extremely clear and readable explanation of the acupuncture points, their meanings, and their uses in bee venom therapy for Lyme and related co-infections.

And the beauty part is – and I say this as an English professor and writer – her latest book, like its predecessors, is a really good read! I know I curled up on a comfortable divan with a cup of coffee and a copy of *Pioneers.* And I certainly look forward to doing the same when the workbook comes out. Just as I would urge my students to immerse themselves in a great novel by Tolstoy, Proust, Joyce, or Faulkner, so I urge everyone I know to make herself at home in Amber Rose's books – and in Amber Rose's world. Who knows? This could be the beginning of a beautiful friendship! And a beautiful healing!

Barry Fruchter, Ph.D.
Associate Professor
English and Latin American Studies, SUNY

INTRODUCTION

DR. AMBER ROSE, PIONEER

There is an expression in Chinese that says, " When drinking water, remember the source." It is often used in martial arts and I have heard it several times in the acupuncture community. It carries the idea that when we are learning a new skill we should take a minute to reflect on the source of the information. So, I am honored to illuminate readers to the source of this knowledge.

It is important to know that Dr. Rose embodies all the traits of a modern saint. By following a healthy combination of her head and her heart she amassed a wealth of knowledge that is only outweighed by her compassion. While her story could fill the pages of an amazing novel, for sake of brevity, we will only cover some highlights.

At an early age our author, teacher, and friend was unhappy with her birth name and in an act of pre-destiny she chose the name Amber Rose. While this act seems to lack much significance at first glance, it is useful to know that the patron saint of beekeepers is St. Ambrose.

In order to explore, understand, and alleviate the suffering of others, Dr. Rose earned advanced degrees in both psychology and theology. Her quest to help improve the health of others continued by earning a degree in acupuncture. This knowledge base would have allowed her to help countless people better their lives and ease their suffering, but as the universe would have it, she was steered into a direction that would allow her to help even more.

After some tough times in her life, including an abusive relationship and some major accidents, the simple act of picking up a Washington Post pointed Dr. Rose to a world where she could not only heal herself, but help others do the same. It was an article about a woman who was treating MS by stinging herself and others with bees. Something resonated with Amber very deeply. The next day she met with this woman to have her first stinging session.

With pain fleeing and hope back in her life, Amber quickly realized that combining her new found love of bees and bee venom therapy (BVT) with her knowledge of acupuncture could offer others a synergistic effect. Within a very small window of time Dr. Rose went from being a patient to treating patients nearly non-stop. Often times she was running a sort of "drive-thru" clinic, where many patients with mobility issues would drive up and Dr. Rose would perform the treatment while the patient stayed in the vehicle. She called it McBees.

Amber firmly believes that bees and BVT are gifts from God and for years performed treatments without charge at her free clinic. She has truly led a life of service.

Some time after combining acupuncture and apitherapy, Dr. Rose took a trip to China to discover that this technique had been around for thousands of years. The problem for much of the world outside of BVT practitioners in China is that there was no extensive knowledge base of this technique. Certainly, there was no way for westerners and those who weren't trained in Oriental Medicine to even have a chance at receiving "Bee-Acupuncture." Amber Rose made it her lifelong mission to change that.

For over 22 years she has been stinging thousands upon thousands of people and helping them recover from very serious conditions including rheumatoid arthritis, multiple sclerosis, and Lyme disease. Dr. Rose has developed a protocol that is in balance with western research, eastern principles, and good common sense. She has published three books that show her mastery and understanding of BVT and acupuncture. The pinnacle of her knowledge is her book, **Bee in Balance**, which has been revised and updated with more information and research. Many apitherapists and acupuncturists worldwide consider this work to be the bible of "Bee - Acupuncture." In fact, there are copies for the first run of this book on sale throughout the internet for hundreds and thousands of dollars apiece. She lectures constantly about BVT and is never too tired to answer a question or help someone begin their own personal health journey.

As a student of hers, although it has been over 15 years since seeing her in person, I can say that being in her presence, one can feel her compassion and universal love. Reading her books and articles, listening to her lectures, and communicating with her via social media immediately fills me with grace, healing, and love.

It brings me great joy to know that Dr. Amber Rose has decided to share this information with you all in a simplified format that is readily accessible.

I am a better acupuncturist and person for knowing Dr. Rose and I'm honored to make this introduction.

Tom Ingegno MSOM, LAc
Licensed Acupuncturist

"For all the beings ailing in the world,

Until their sickness has been healed,

May I become the doctor and the cure,

And may I nurse them back to health."

　　　Shantideva Bodhicaryāvatāra—

　　　Chapter 3, Verse 8

CHAPTER 1

THE PHILOSOPHY OF ORIENTAL MEDICINE:
THE BASIC LAWS OF ACUPUNCTURE

All true healing comes from nature. Five thousand years ago, the ancient Chinese believed that the world was made up of five basic elements: wood, fire, earth, metal, and water. These correspond to the seasons of the year and the seasons within us. Each of us was knocked off balance somewhere in childhood on one of these elements and never quite recovered.

The ancient Chinese developed acupuncture as a method of bringing the body back into balance. They believed that all sickness was due to an imbalance in the body, mind, and spirit. Their basic goal was to restore balance and maintain harmony. They did this by removing blocks that prevent the free flow of energy in the body. Then the body heals itself. Traditional acupuncture treats the whole person, not just the symptoms.

According to ancient oriental philosophy, every human being is part of nature. Each one of us is a miniature cosmos, a replica of the great cosmos (that is nature). We are each unique in our own way and yet we are the same. Just like snowflakes: no two are exactly the same and yet they are all snowflakes.

There is an order to nature, but within that order, nature is in a state of constant flux. It is in accordance with this principle that our world is always changing. Nature does her dance, she is our teacher. Nature has her patterns, yet we cannot count on anything to remain the same.

 Ancient wisdom says, "Change is the only truth in the universe" and "there is nothing permanent but change." The weather changes, the seasons change, and so, we too, must be open to change. When we stop growing or we resist change, we are more likely to get sick. We must keep our bodies in a relaxed and open state to keep energy flowing. We must follow the way of the Tao. Tao refers to the whole of life, and your path within it.

PATHWAYS AND THE FLOW OF CH'I

Acupuncture is a branch of Oriental Medicine which assists the healing process by using needles to either stimulate (tonify) or calm (sedate) specific points along pathways of energy which are called meridians.These meridians are not anatomically distinct, but have been discovered by the Chinese through centuries of experience and a sensitivity to the flow of life energy. This energy flows through this series of channels in an orderly flow that assists the body in maintaining harmony.

There are 12 major meridians which are bilateral, meaning that they flow along both sides of the body. The location of the pathway and its points is symmetrical. This book also describes points on two extra meridians, which are found at the front and rear center line of the body and are not bilateral.

The Chinese discovered that illness in the body, mind, or spirit is often accompanied by blocks in the flow of this energy. These blocks can be alleviated in many circumstances by using needles or bees to "direct" the energy in a way that restores the smooth flow of energy. Acupuncturists also use a technique called Moxibustion, in which heat is added to the point, similar to the heat of the bee venom.

The energy of the life force we are talking about is called "Ch'i" or "Qi" by the Chinese. This energy flows through the meridians. The Chinese character for Ch'i is a cooking vessel filled with rice. Steam is coming out of it. The Ch'i is not even the steam but the essence of the steam. Ch'i is considered to be totally non-physical.

The points along the meridians are openings into the flow of Ch'i which allow a needle, or a honeybee sting, to affect the quality of Ch'i in the meridian. This is where you can gain access to the person. Each point has its own unique function or "spirit." The art of acupuncture is to determine the changes in energy flow needed and what points to use to bring about those changes.

This is done first by a series of cleansings to clear blockages, by balancing treatments on the element(s) most out of balance, and then by using seasonal points and "spirit points." The names of certain acupuncture points (Spirit Burial Ground, Greater Mountain Stream, Spirit Path, and Joining the Valleys) call forth a need to return to the earth, while other points (Windows of the Sky, Soul Door, and Utmost Source) speak to our yearning to reach for the sky and touch the stars.

Each person is given the opportunity for a personal vision quest through acupuncture, so that they may experience the alchemy of turning their suffering into gold.

YIN/YANG

In oriental philosophy the principle that the world is always changing is known as the Law of Yin/Yang. Life takes place in the alternating rhythm of yin and yang. There is a continual interchange and communication between the two. Day gives way to night and night to day. There is a cold, dark side of the mountain (yin) and a warm, sunny side of the mountain (yang). Everything has an inside (yin) and an outside (yang), a top (yang) and a bottom (yin). Flowers open (yang) and close (yin).

Yin and yang are like an inseparable couple. Their proper and balanced relationship is healthy, while a disturbance in their relationship is disease. If you look at the yin/yang symbol you will see a small black dot within the white area. This is the yin within the yang. The white dot in the black area is the yang within the yin. Nothing is pure yin or yang. Each has a small seed of the other. Everything has the possibility of turning into its opposite.

THE LAW OF THE FIVE ELEMENTS

A central understanding in the Chinese view of healing flows directly from the yin/yang principle. The tension between yin and yang creates five phases or elements. The Chinese saw the world as composed of wood, fire, earth, metal (air),and water. These elements follow the order of the five seasons of nature: spring, summer, late summer, autumn, and winter.

3

The five elements are as different from each other as five different notes on a scale. Therefore, the five seasons have five different qualities. Spring is very different from autumn and summer is nothing like winter. Each of the five elements has correspondences that go with it. Each element has a color, a season, a taste, an odor, a sound, an organ, a time of day, etc., associated with it. Each element also has an emotion associated with it. Anger (the emotion that goes with the spring and the wood element) feels very different from joy (the emotion that goes with the summer and the fire element). So, as you can see, each element is distinctly different from the other elements. But each one has an effect on the others. In brief, people who have a particular element out of balance will feel the following:

When the wood element is out of balance, the person may feel angry, frustrated, impatient, and confused. This person needs a plan, a sense of direction, and hope.

When the fire element is out of balance, the person may be depressed, lack joy, or appear cold and distant. This kind of person needs warmth, unconditional love, and joy.

When the earth element is out of balance, the person may worry a lot or have a need to take care of others (perhaps always putting others before themselves). This person is going to need compassion, sympathy, and to be understood.

When the metal element is out of balance, the person may be stuck in guilt, grief, loss, emptiness, or negative thinking. This type of patient needs to be respected, appreciated, and to feel that life has meaning.

When the water element is out of balance, the patient may have a great deal of fear. This person needs reassurance that everything is going to be OK. The person needs to feel powerful and courageous.

Shen Cycle: This chart depicts the Shen cycle, or the cycle of creation, in which each element gives birth to the next one. Each element is the mother of the next. Understanding the clockwise flow and the order in which each element is the mother to the next is central to understanding the Law of the Five Elements.

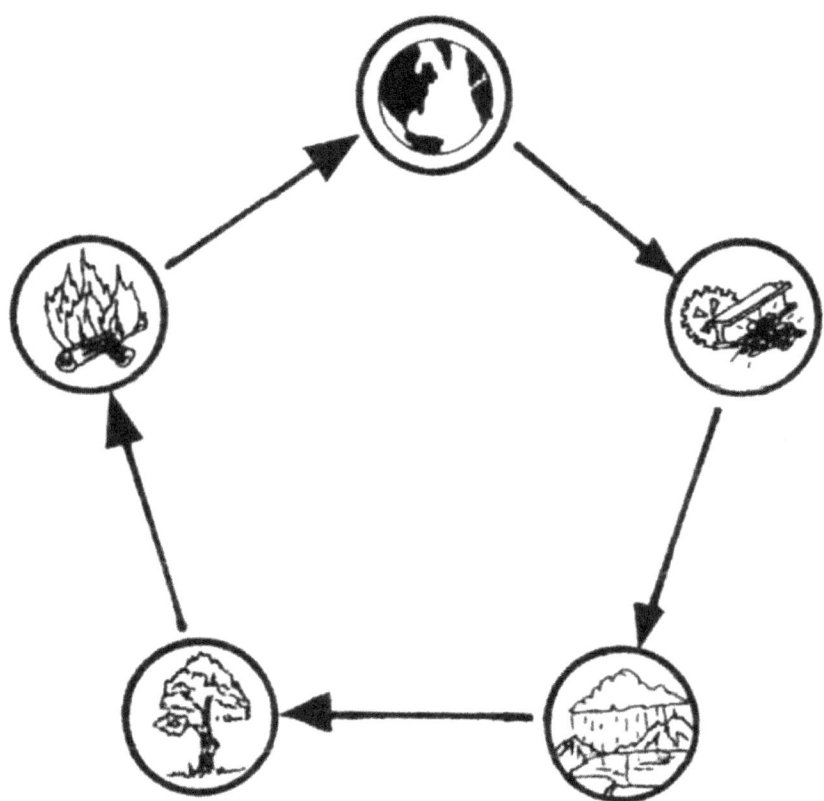

Shen: The Cycle of Creation

Health and disease result from the quality and the flow of life energy. There are two major kinds of relationships (or cycles) within the five elements: the creation cycle and the control cycle. In the creation cycle, also called the Sheng or the Shen cycle, the energy flows from one meridian or pathway to the next in the order described in the accompanying Shen chart. The energy in this creation cycle flows in a clockwise direction around the circle. The flow is continuous. The cycle of energy has no beginning and no end. The five elements are inseparable. You can't have one without the others. Each element gives birth to the next one on the cycle. This brings us the Law of Mother and Son. Since one element gives birth to the next one on the cycle wood is the mother of fire, and fire is the son of wood, and so on around the circle.

The flow of Shen can be thought of in this manner:

WOOD CREATES FIRE Two pieces of wood together can produce a spark.

FIRE CREATES EARTH Fire transforms burning matter into ashes.

EARTH CREATES METAL Within the earth, metal (ore) is buried.

METAL CREATES WATER Metal becomes a liquid when it melts.

WATER CREATES WOOD A tree cannot grow without water.

This concept becomes important for purposes of diagnosis, because sometimes the element that is the "child" has more symptoms than the "mother" element. Now, what this means in terms of dis-ease is that if the fire element is out of balance (or "sick") then the earth element will be struggling as well, because it's getting either too much or too little energy from its mother, fire. In the Law of Mother and Son, we often notice that the son may cry out louder than the mother. When the fire element is out of balance, for example, you might get a lot of symptoms in the earth element. You may be tempted to treat the earth. If the real problem is that the fire element is out of balance, treating the earth element may only give you temporary relief. This is because you are treating the symptoms (the child) and not the root cause (the mother). On the other hand, let's say you have a lot of symptoms on the fire element. It's possible that the earth element is really the first one that went out of balance and you're getting symptoms in the fire element because it's the mother of the earth. In this case, treating the symptoms (fire), will be less successful than treating the root cause (the earth). The reason I am mentioning this is that if you decide to work on a certain element first and you don't get the desired results, you may want to treat the element either before it or after it on the five element cycle.

If a mother does not have enough milk or if she is too weak to take care of her child, the baby may start to cry. Let's say we hear the baby crying. So we go into the room and pick up the crying child. The child may stop crying for a while, but we must also help the mother. If we don't, then sooner or later, after we put the child down, it will begin to cry again. This is the best argument I know for not just treating symptoms. The cause of the symptoms may be coming from someplace else. You could end up chasing symptoms forever.

Going back to our analogy, we may need to support the mother and reconnect her with the child. Therefore, we may have to treat the fire element before we treat the earth element. I realize it may be very tempting to treat the earth element first, because it has more symptoms, but I strongly encourage you to try and identify the cause of the problem, not just the symptoms. I will explain this in more detail as we go on.

The Mother/Son relationship does not go backwards, because the energy of the creation cycle only moves in a clockwise direction. For example, if a child is hungry, you bring the mother to the child and give him the mother's breast. This is assuming the mother is strong and there is enough milk. But if the mother is hungry or weak, you don't give her the child to eat. So, in other words the cycle does not go backwards; earth does not give to fire. This would be like the child taking care of the mother and that is not the way it is supposed to be. That is out of balance. That would be a dysfunctional family; as a mother should not have a son in order to be loved, so the element which is the "son" should not take care of the "mother."

K'o Cycle: The Dance of Control

This energy brings us to the second kind of relationship within the five elements, the K'o or control cycle. The balance of energy in the body is maintained not only by Shen's creating and feeding the next element, but by K'o's limitation of the energy through control. Water is the mother of wood and wood is the mother of fire; therefore water is the grandmother of fire. This relationship of checks and balances is called the K'o cycle and this feedback cycle helps keep the Ch'i in balance. The grandmother controls the grandchild by her presence, just by being there. For example, the presence of water holds fire in check. If there is too much water, it will put out the fire. Water, which is the grandmother of the fire, will keep excessive fire in balance. This is not a flow of energy like the creation cycle. It is not feeding the fire; but regulating its intensity.

This control can become destructive if it becomes overbearing. When the K'o cycle is in a state of imbalance it becomes a destructive cycle:

WOOD DESTROYS EARTH - The tree begins to suck strength from the earth.

EARTH DESTROYS WATER - Earth can halt the flow of water (like a dam). Earth can soak up too much water (like a mud slide).

WATER DESTROYS FIRE - Water will extinguish or put out the flame.

FIRE DESTROYS METAL - Fire will cause metal to melt.

METAL DESTROYS WOOD - The axe can cut down the tree.

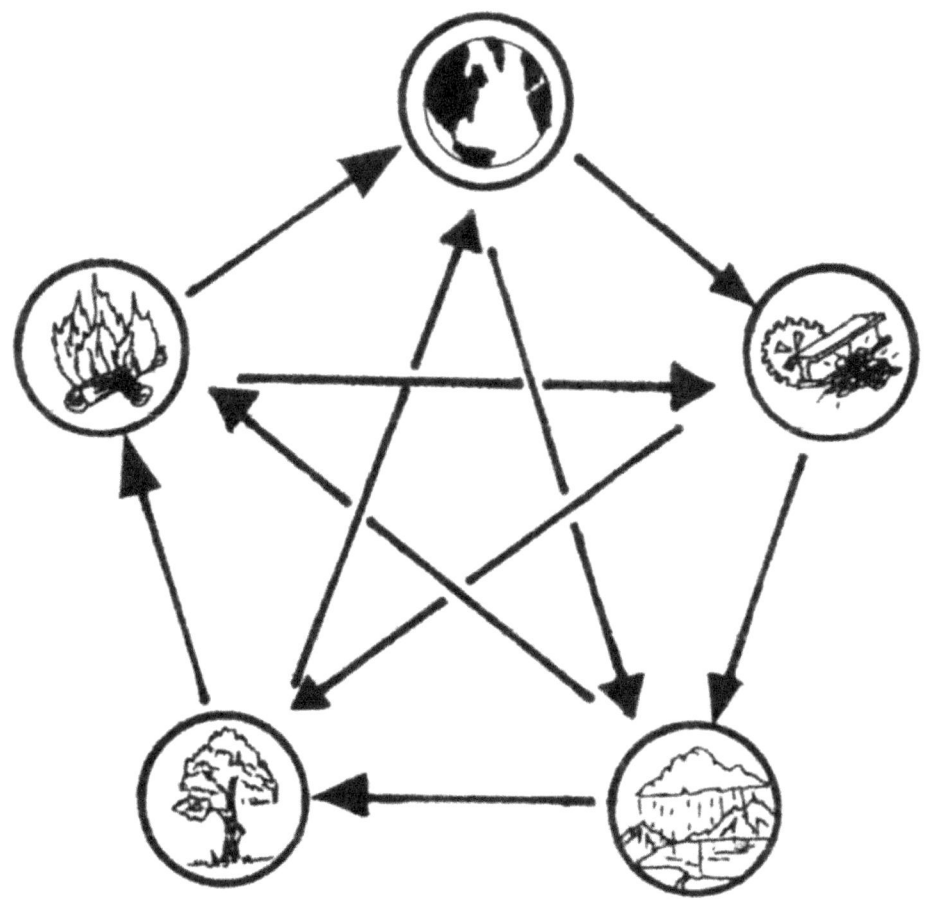

Shen and K'o Cycle: This chart shows the K'o cycle in addition to the Shen cycle. The five-sided star shows the path of the K'o cycle. You can see from this chart that fire is the grandmother of metal according to the K'o cycle, and the mother of earth,
according to the Shen cycle.

Another way to understand the K'o cycle is to see the relationships between the elements in this way:

Wood is the grandmother of earth

Earth is the grandmother of water

Water is the grandmother of fire

Fire is the grandmother of metal

Metal is the grandmother of wood

Just as I mentioned in discussing the Shen cycle, there are times when you may need to treat an element which precedes the element that you've chosen as needing the most attention. In the Shen cycle, that would be the mother. There may be times when you want to follow the path of the K'o cycle and tonify or strengthen the grandmother of the element you are working on. For example, if the element in which your primary issues arise is too strong, you may be able to sedate it by tonifying the grandmother. This would result in the grandmother increasing her control over the grandson and thus reducing the grandson's energy. If, instead, the element you're focusing on is lacking in energy, you may want to sting the son in addition to the element itself. You will note that the son is the grandmother of the grandmother, so that this treatment follows the K'o cycle—tonifying the great-great grandmother tempers the grandmother, thus allowing the original deficient element the freedom to increase.

Bee stings are a potent way to tonify or strengthen a pathway or point. Because bee stings are highly energizing, they cannot be used to sedate a point or a pathway; this is a technique which requires the skilled use of acupuncture needles. If you believe that sedating a pathway is an important approach, you may want to consider tonifying the grandmother as described above.

Excessive control can eventually bring about a condition called Aggressive Energy. (Some people call this: Clearing Jaki.)This imbalance is considered one of the major blocks; these blocks and their treatments are discussed in the chapter on Major Blocks. If you find yourself pulled between very high energy states and serious depression, this could be due to an imbalance in which excessive energy in one part of your system dampens energy in another. Such swings in mood or energy level might be treated by both addressing the K'o cycle and by draining Aggressive Energy. Some people's focus on a particular area—in which they may either excel or obsess—can cause other areas in their life to suffer. If the elements you choose in the following chapter have a grandmother-son relationship, then you may want to consider the K'o cycle as you choose the pathways to sting.

THE CAUSATIVE FACTOR

Treating the Cause and not the Symptoms

In addition to all the blocks that can develop along the way on our own journey to wholeness, a trained classical acupuncturist will be looking to see where each person was originally knocked off balance in childhood. This could have been something like pneumonia, a high fever, or even a death in the family. This original imbalance or illness is called the causative factor (CF). It is the first element that went out of balance and stayed out of balance. This will be the weak link in the chain, the one most likely to go under stress. The CF is where you can go to gain access to the person in treatment and everything else changes.

I need to emphasize here, that it is very difficult, or perhaps impossible, to diagnose a patient's CF from reading a book. A trained acupuncturist can make such a determination, and then only with a face to face consultation with the person. Such a diagnosis is based on a myriad of considerations, such as the color on the face, the sound of the voice, the smell of the body, and from a sense as to which emotion is most out of balance. The goal of this book is not to help you definitively arrive at the CF, but to help you see which element may be most out of balance for you. This gives you a good place to focus your treatment.

Imagine that each person is like a desert. Now think about this: what can I bring to this person that will make the biggest difference? If I bring plants (wood) to a desert, it will not change anything. If I bring more heat (fire) to a desert, it will not make a difference. If I bring more dirt (earth) to a desert, nothing changes. If I bring metal (air) to the desert, it stays the same. But, if I bring water to the desert, it will change everything! And it's the same way with people. You need to decide which element will make the biggest difference to the person. It is usually the element that was the first one to be knocked off balance.

11

Please keep in mind that it may not be the element that is "screaming" the loudest or has the most symptoms.

The decision as to which element is the primary one or the CF is totally based on the color, the sound, the odor and the emotion. That is why it is hard to diagnose yourself from a book. The CF is only truly diagnosed by a trained acupuncturist who is able to see the patient.

Understanding the balance of energy in the body, where distortions and blocks have become ingrained, and which are primary, helps you get to the root of the problem. You need to get to the root cause and not just treat on the surface. If you think of a person as a tree, you must treat the roots and not just the branches. If you nourish the roots the branches will become healthy again. If you just treat the branches you can't help the whole tree.

Classical acupuncture aims to get to the root cause. The body is seen as a dynamic whole, a network of interacting energies. So, if you support the place where the person was originally knocked off balance, the body will heal itself and the symptoms will disappear on their own. As in the domino theory, if you tap the first domino, all the others fall on their own.

Let's take another example. Look at your car. If the oil light in your car is flashing, you wouldn't want the mechanic to cut the wire. Although it would prevent the light from flashing, you would rather the mechanic get down to the root cause, wouldn't you? Where your health is concerned, even more than for your car, you'd certainly want someone to be able to find the root cause of your condition and not just cover up the problem. Although it is tempting to go for the quick fix, I believe in my heart that we all truly want to be healed from the inside and not just on the surface.

Any illness invites us home to take a moment to sift through levels of our experience and be open to needed changes. When illness arises we must stop, look, and listen. When we experience dis-ease a message is trying to come through which we haven't received yet. This message will persist, increasing in intensity and frequency, until we see it. We can choose to be open to it, to avoid it, or even hate it. Any resistance can create a conflict or struggle and this will determine the degree of our illness. Remember, all sickness is homesickness. We are all Dorothys and Totos from "The Wizard of Oz." We are all just trying to find our way home again, home to ourselves.

THE CHINESE CLOCK

Every 24 hours the Ch'i flows through the whole body via the 12 main meridians. Each meridian is at its peak for two hours, and 12 hours later it will be at its lowest point. This is called the Law of Midday-Midnight or the Law of the Chinese Clock.

The theory behind the Chinese Clock can give you very valuable information for understanding yourself and others. If there is a weakness, excess, or block on one of the pathways, you may get symptoms at the same time every day. Patients may make comments like this:

"I'm always tired in the late afternoon."
"I am not a morning person."
"I am a night person."

You can take advantage of this clock. By treating a pathway when it is at its peak, you can get a more powerful response. This can be increased even more by treating the meridian at the right time of day in the right season. This is called a horary treatment. A horary treatment is done by treating the home element point—the point on that pathway which is the same element as the pathway, i.e., a wood point on a wood pathway.

Let's say you want to strengthen the heart pathway. The time of day for the heart meridian is 11 a.m.-1 p.m. So you would have your patient come to see you at that time of day. And it's even better if they can come in at that time of day in the summer, because that is the season that goes with the heart. Since the heart is part of the fire element, you will want to treat the fire point on that pathway. That is what I meant when I said that you will treat the home element point on the pathway. If you were treating a wood pathway, you would be looking for the

13

wood point on the wood pathway. Another name for a home element point is a horary point. There is only one horary point on each pathway.

The Chinese Clock: Because the energy moves through all twelve meridians in a 24-hour day, each pathway is at its peak for two hours. If a particular pathway is deficient, you may feel better during the time of day of that pathway. If a pathway has excess energy, then your symptoms may intensify during that time of day. For example, someone with deficient energy in the heart may feel better around lunch time. Someone with excess energy in the liver may be unable to sleep between 1 a.m. and 3 a.m. The times on this chart refer to "sun-time." During daylight savings time, be sure to subtract an hour.

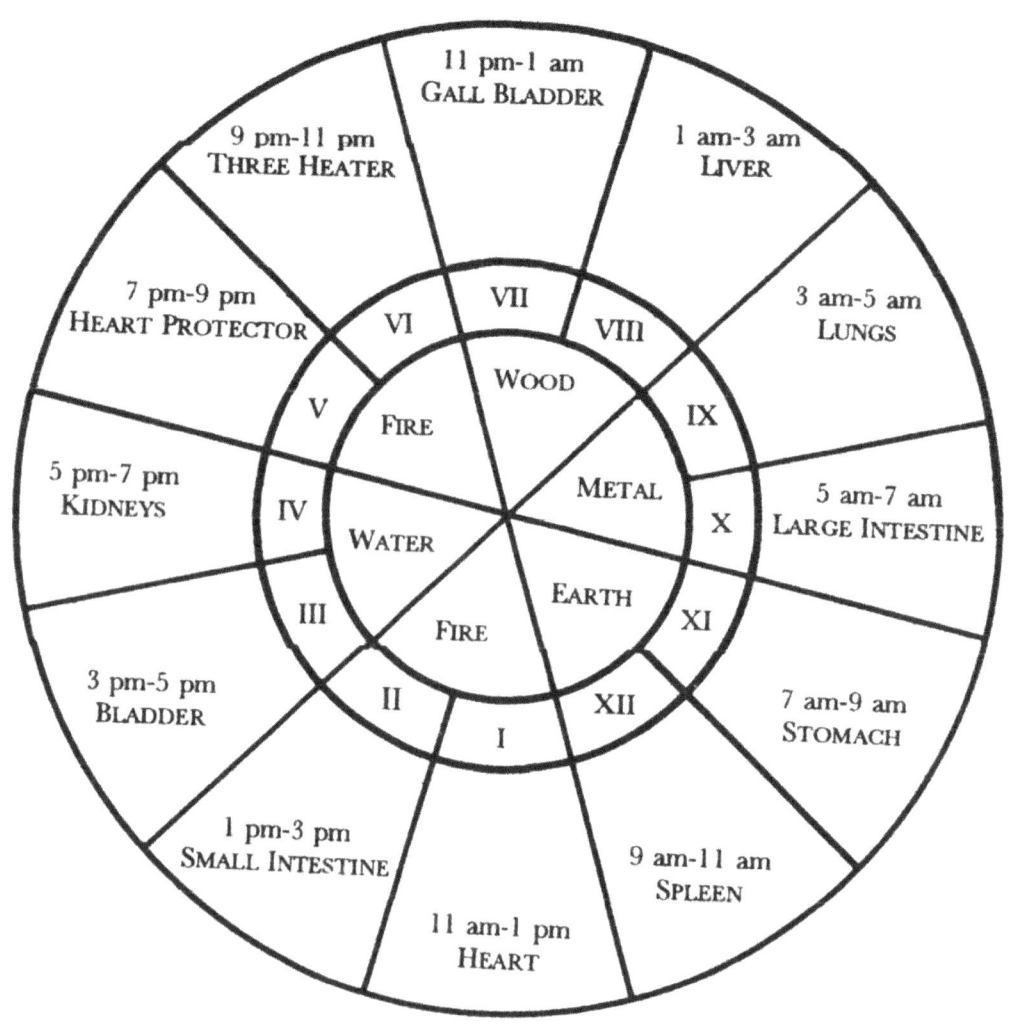

FINDING YOURSELF WITHIN THE FIVE ELEMENTS

Please circle or underline any symptoms listed on the next two pages that relate to you. When you are all done, you will be ready to select which one of the five elements (wood, fire, earth, metal, or water) seems the most out of balance for you. Consider the seriousness of the symptoms selected in each element as well as the number. This will suggest the element that you turn to first. At this point you will turn to the section that goes with that element. For example, if you have

15

chosen to work with the Wood element first, then turn to the chapter entitled Manifestations of the Wood Element. You will then continue to underline the characteristics that relate to you.

Some diseases are thought to primarily manifest themselves in a particular element. The Chinese believe, for example, that MS, arthritis, and other chronic diseases can often be treated on the earth . . . spleen and stomach, and the wood   . . . gall bladder and liver pathways. Each element is affected by a particular climate; the earth is affected by dampness, the wood, affected by wind. The Chinese believe that dampness and wind have invaded the body to produce what they consider to be rheumatoid conditions—MS, arthritis, and other similar chronic diseases. It is important, though, to learn to understand each individual person. As Hippocrates said, it's more important to treat the person with the disease than the disease. Only in this way can you get to the underlying cause and treat the whole picture.

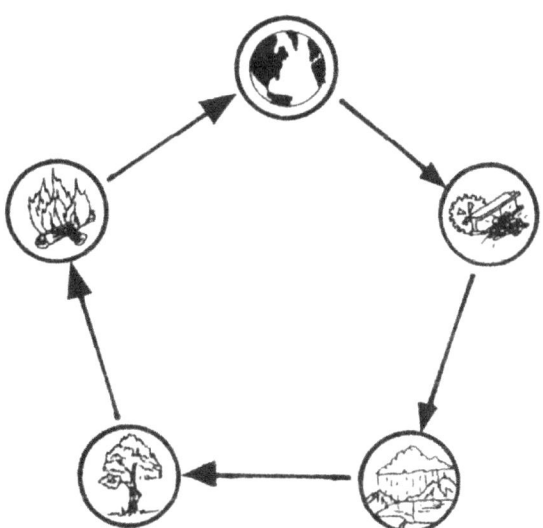

Circle each symptom you experience listed for each of the five elements—then determine which element you appear to be having the most trouble with based on the number and severity of the conditions circled. Then turn to the section for that element.

POTENTIAL MANIFESTATIONS
OF IMBALANCES IN THE FIVE ELEMENTS:

WOOD

Liver or gall bladder problems, hepatitis, jaundice, allergies, migraines, headaches(either one-sided or headaches that feel like a tight band around the head); problems with tendons and ligaments, lack of coordination, MS, fibromyalgia; migrating pains (pains that move around), dry or brittle nails/nail biting, chronic fatigue syndrome or Epstein-Barre; eye problems; anger, irritability, impatience, frustration, needing a sense of direction, trouble making decisions, procrastination, addictions; a creative person, artists, singers, dancers, writers; likes or dislikes spring, green, sour taste; may be a night person or may wake up or have trouble sleeping between 11 p.m. and 3 a.m.

FIRE

High fevers (especially in childhood, i.e., rheumatic fever, scarlet fever, measles), issues with hot and cold; heart problems, circulatory problems; small intestine problems; sexual problems or sexual abuse; fibromyalgia; stuttering, feelings of chaos and panic, issues of control (fear of being around a controlling person, needing to be in control, feeling out of control), feeling "spacey" or confused, can't sort things out, has too many options and doesn't know what to do, "absent-minded professor," issues of trust, fear of being hurt/rejected, feeling unloved, relationship issues, wanting unconditional love, feeling responsible for everyone else (like the conductor of an orchestra, "if I'm not taking care of things, everything falls apart"); likes or dislikes summer, red, bitter tastes, may use humor a lot or laugh a lot, "class clown," "comedian," or a lack of laughter and joy; trouble falling asleep; issues between 11 a.m. and 3p.m. and 7 p.m. and 11 p.m.

EARTH

Stomach and spleen problems, digestive troubles, vomiting, nausea, belching, burping, hiatal hernias, ulcers, anorexia/bulimia; lumps, cysts, (especially breast); spinning and dizziness, craving sweets, diabetes or low blood sugar, pancreas

17

problems; leg cramps, muscle problems, MS, feeling very tired and heavy, (like a slug—just can't move, "I just can't get out of this chair I can't even lift my arm"), chronic fatigue syndrome; overweight or unusual distribution of weight; obsessions, "poor me," never satisfied, not feeling centered or grounded, nightmares, smothering someone else or fear of being smothered emotionally, feeling needy, wanting sympathy, needing to be understood or feeling misunderstood, a caretaker or wanting to be taken care of, issues around mothering, nurturing and your relationship with your own mother; likes or dislikes the color yellow, sweets, humidity, "a morning person" or dislikes the morning; issues between 7 a.m. and 11 a.m.

METAL

Lung problems (especially in childhood), bronchitis, pneumonia, pleurisy, asthma, allergies, coughs, sore throats, mononucleosis, leukemia, environmental illness; large intestine problems, diarrhea, spastic colon, constipation, hernia, excess mucus, skin problems; difficulties with the nose or sense of smell, sinus problems, headaches; feeling cut-off and alone, fear of being alone and a need for connections, or a loner, low self-esteem and self-worth, wears excess metal jewelry; issues with your relationship with your father or your heavenly father; searching for father substitute/mentor/guru; likes vacations to the mountains, helped by meditation, tends to focus on the negative, complains a lot, the wailing wall syndrome, living in the past, sadness and unresolved grief and loss (divorces, deaths, moving to a new area—the loss of friends or support system), perfectionism, judgmental and unforgiving, has trouble letting go, can never throw anything out or likes to keep things very clean; likes or dislikes autumn, white, spicy foods, dryness; may wake up between 3 a.m. and 7 a.m., or have dreams of sharp objects, flying, death and dying.

WATER

Bladder and kidney problems, spine problems, spinal meningitis, brain problems, epilepsy; combination of low back and knee problems, blood pressure issues, teeth problems, excess perspiration, ear disorders; environmental illness; feeling burnt out, wants a vacation (especially to the water); fear, anxiety, panic attacks, fear of bridges, darkness, claustrophobia, lack of fear, feeling overwhelmed, no ambition/will; afraid of bees, spiders, and other insects; likes or dislikes winter, the cold, salty foods, the color blue or black, issues between 3 p.m. and 7 p.m.

Continue on – all the way through Chapter 2. And even if you feel you have answered these questions before, answer them again with fresh eyes and ears: listen to that small, still voice inside you. This is the heart and soul of this workbook.

CHAPTER 2

5 ELEMENT QUESTIONNAIRE & QUESTIONS

Name_____ Date_____

Address_____ Birth date_____

City_____ State_____

Zipcode_____

Phone (home)_____cell phone_____

Children:
Name   age

Major health problems

_____
_____
_____
_____
_____
_____
_____

Is your father alive?   If not, what was the cause of death?
_____

Does he/did he have any other major health problems? Describe.

_____
_____

Is your mother alive?   If not, what was the cause of death?
_____

_____

Does she/did she have any other major health problems? Describe.

_____

_____

Brothers and sisters:

Name   age

Major health problems

_____

_____

_____

_____

Do you feel close to your family?

_____

_____

What is/was your occupation?

_____

_____

What do you do when you're not at work?

_____

_____

_____

Why have you come for treatment?

_____

_____

_____

_____

How long have you had this problem?

_____

What have you done about it?

_____

_____

_____

What would your life be like if you didn't have this problem?

_____

_____

_____

_____

Is there anything else that is important that you want to mention or anything else you need help with?

_____

Medical history: childhood illnesses:

_____

_____

_____

Major/serious illnesses:

_____

_____

_____

_____

_____

Physical or emotional traumas

_____

_____

_____

_____

_____

_____

Surgeries/hospitalizations/scars_____

Other memories that stand out?

_____
_____
_____
_____

What are your normal sleeping hours?

_____

Do you sleep well?_____Do you wake up at night? If so when?

_____
_____

What do you dream about?

_____
_____

How is your appetite?_____What is your diet like?

_____
_____

What kinds of fluids do you drink?

_____
_____

Do you drink alcohol? If so, how much?

_____

Are your bowels regular?_____

Do you have difficulty with urination?

_____

Do you perspire normally?_____Do you get cold hands and feet?

_____

Do you feel that your sexual energy is high, low or normal?_____

_____

For women only:
How old were you when you first started your period?_____

Have you experienced pain, cramping, bloating or mood swings?_____

Have you reached menopause?_____What symptoms have you had?

_____

_____

Method of contraception?_____

Have you ever smoked?_____Do you smoke now?

Are you taking any medication? If so, what kind?

_____

_____

Have you ever had hepatitis?_____

Have you been exposed to HIV/AIDS?

What is your favorite season?_____What is your worst season?_____

What is your favorite time of day? (be specific)

_____

What is your worst time of day? (be specific)

_____

_____

Do you have symptoms at the same time every day? If so, what are they?

_____

_____

_____

_____

What is your favorite climate?_____What is your worst climate?_____Which do you prefer, humidity or dryness?_____

What is your favorite color?_____What is your worst color?

_____

What is your favorite taste: sour, bitter, sweet,

Spicy or salty? _____

What is your worst taste: sour, bitter, sweet, spicy

Or salty?_____

If you could wave a magic wand, what do you really need right now?_____

_____

THE FIVE IMPORTANT QUESTIONS:

Which of the following is the most important to you:

1. Being loved unconditionally?_____

2. Feeling understood?_____

3. Feeling respected and appreciated?_____

4. Feeling reassured that everything is going to be ok?_____

5. Having a sense of direction?

The Fire Element:

Is unconditional love the most important thing

   in the world to you?

Are you happy? Do you feel loved?

Do you have enough friends/love in your life?

Do you like or dislike the color red?

Do you dream about fire/people/relationships?

Did you have a high fever in childhood?

Do you have a good sense of humor?

Do you like to laugh and makes jokes?

Were you ever involved in an actual fire or lightning strike?

Like or dislike of heat/summer?

Filled with joy or lack of joy?

Like or dislike bitter foods?

Specific Fire Meridians

The Heart:

Do you have any heart problems? High fevers in childhood: scarlet

fever, rheumatic fever, heart murmurs, history of electric shocks

or lightning strike?

Do you have trouble falling asleep?

Do you feel overly responsible (like the conductor

of an orchestra)…do you have trouble

delegating responsibility or feel like: if you don't

do it, it doesn't get done?

Do you have issues with control? Needing to be in

control? Or not liking it if others are in control?

Is insight and wisdom one of your strengths?

Recurring issues from 11am – 1pm?

Feelings of failure?

Insomnia or anxiety??

The Small Intestine:

Do you ever feel like an absent-minded professor?

Are you a "space cadet"? Very spacey??

Do you have trouble or get confused when you

have too many options??

Trouble distinguishing between self & other?

Issues between 1pm – 3pm?

The Heart Protector /Pericardium:

Do you often feel vulnerable? Do you need to

feel safe?

Has your heart been broken recently?

Do you get hurt or embarrassed easily?

History of rape or sexual abuse or incest?

Do you have issues with trust/betrayal/intimacy?

Do you believe in love?

Do you have some issues with sexuality or

circulation?

Issues between 7-9pm?

Palpitations?

The Three Heater:

Is having fun very important to you? Are you the

life of the party? Or the host/hostess? Were you a "class clown" in

school? Are you a comedian?Are you a networker/peace-maker?

Are you in sales?

Do you consider yourself a "people-person"?

Do you like to receive or give hugs? Are you a

"touchy-feeling" kind of person? Or do you dislike being touched?

Do you have trouble with groups/public speaking?

or do you love speaking in public?

Thermostat issues: too hot and/or too cold?

Issues between 9-11pm

<u>The Earth Element</u>:

How's your appetite? How is your digestion?

Are you a worry-wart?

Are you overweight or underweight?

Are you a caretaker or do you want to be taken

care of?

Are you a morning person?

Is being understood very important to you?

Do you feel like some people just don't understand

you?

Do you like or dislike sweets?

Do you have trouble with humidity? Or do you love it?

How is/was your relationship with your mother?

Do you put other people's needs first, before your

own…and then get lost in the shuffle?

Is it hard for you to ask for help?

Do you like/or dislike cooking, eating?

Do you have nightmares or dreams of houses?

Do you have many ailments that no doctor can

figure out?

History of any lumps, tumors, cysts?

History of blood sugar problems: diabetes or

hypoglycemia? Leg cramps?

Any pregnancy or miscarriage issues…or issues re:

not having children…?

Empty nest syndrome?

Do you have issues of abandonment/nurturing

or feeling smothered?

Do you like or dislike the color yellow and late

summer?

Do you like or dislike singing?

Poor me feelings? Trouble saying no?

Craving empathy & sympathy?

Specific Earth Meridians

Stomach Meridian:

Have you ever had stomach problems: acid reflux,

   a hiatal hernia, or a stomach ulcer, etc.?

Problems/issues from 7 am – 9 am?

Spleen Meridian:

Do you obsess about little things?

Do your legs/arms ever feel heavy?

Do you ever get dry/chapped lips?

Chronic fatigue? Diabetes or pancreas

   issues?

Prolapsed organs, veins?

Nightmares or spinning?

Issues between 9- 11 am?

The Metal Element:

How is your relationship with your father?

Have you had a major loss in your life? When?

Was there anyone in your life who was very

   critical?

How is your self - esteem/ self-worth?

Do you need to be the "Rock of Gibraltar"?

Are you a perfectionist?

Do you like or dislike the mountains?

Do you dream of flying, sharp objects or things

made of metal?

Do you like or dislike the color white?

Do you know what is precious to you?

Do you like to wear jewelry?

How is the quality of your life?

Do you like or dislike spicy foods?

How is your sense of smell?

Do you like or dislike dryness and/or fall?

Is there a sad or weepy sound to your voice?

Do you need respect, appreciation, and to feel special?

Would you consider yourself a spiritual/ religious

person?

Do you meditate, pray, or feel connected to god or

a higher power?

Do you have financial issues or concerns?

Specific Metal Meridians

Lung Meridian:

Any lung problems: i.e. pneumonia, bronchitis,

pleurisy? Have you ever smoked?

Any skin problems? Mucus issues, allergies, sore

throats, mono, leukemia, trouble between 3 –

5am?

Trouble receiving love or feeling empty? Strong

feelings of guilt?

Large Intestine (Colon) Meridian:

Are you a "neat-freak"/ or "a total slob"?

Do you collect things?

Do you ever feel like either you know it all or

you know nothing?

Do you live in the past or complain a lot?

Would you consider yourself a negative person?

Do you have trouble letting go of people, places,

or things? Is it hard for you to forgive yourself

or others? Is feeling connected very important

to you…or do you feel like a loner sometimes…

and therefore cut off from others?

Do you have trouble with your bowels: i.e. either

constipation or diarrhea? IBS? Hernias?

Issues between 5-7am??

The Water Element:

Do you like salty foods? Potato chips? Pretzels?

Do you like cold weather/winter?

Would you consider yourself a fearful person?

Are you a dare-devil?

Do you like to look at water? The ocean? A lake? A

stream or a waterfall? Does it feel soothing/

peaceful?

Do you have any phobias?(fear of the dark? Insects?)

How are your teeth? Any broken bones?

Have you had any kidney/bladder or prostate

problems?

Do you need reassurance that everything is going

to be ok?

Do you like or dislike the color blue or black?

Do you feel refreshed if you take a nap, especially

between 3pm and 7pm?

Do you dream about water/ice?

<u>Specific Water Meridians</u>

<u>Bladder Meridian:</u>

Have you ever had sciatica?

Do you often feel burnt out, burning your candle

at both ends?

If you feel tired, does it feel like somebody just

"pulled the plug"?

Do you sometimes feel like you are the energizer

bunny and you have lots of energy?

Do you feel overwhelmed and feel like you need a

vacation?

Issues between 3-5pm?

<u>Kidney Meridian</u>:

Do you feel brave or courageous?

Do you have low back and/or knee pain???

Were you born with any congenital problems?

Any spine or brain injuries?

Do you have scary dreams? Or sexual dreams?

35

How is your willpower?

Do you have much ambition?

Any issues between 5-7pm

The Wood Element:

Do you experience a lot of anger?

Are you easily frustrated, impatient, or irritable?

Do you like or dislike sour foods?

Do you enjoy or dislike spring?

Do you like or dislike the wind?

Do you have aches and pains that migrate (move around

 your body)?

Do you have headaches very often??

Do you ever get migraines? Floaters? Eye problems?

Are you a night person?

Do you have any problems sleeping between 11pm

 and 3am?

Do you feel like you need a sense of direction?

Are you an artist, writer, dancer, musician, or poet?

Do you feel envious or jealous of other people?

Does the grass always seem greener somewhere

else? Do you like/dislike the color green?

Specific Wood Meridians

Gall Bladder Meridian:

If you have headaches …are they one sided or

temporal?

Do you tend to procrastinate a lot??

Do you make lists? Do you pay attention to details?

Do you know how to make your dreams come

true?

Do you have trouble making decisions?

Any specific gall bladder problems?

Any specific shoulder problems? Or any one-sided problems?

Do you have trouble with ligaments/ tendons? Or hip pain?

Does life seem unfair or unjust? Are you a crusader

for justice?

Issues between 11pm-1am?

Liver meridian:

If you have headaches… do they feel like a tight hat-

band or like your head is in a vise?

Can you see the future? The big picture? Dreams & goals?

Do you ever feel hopeless or lost?

Any involvement with drugs/alcohol or

trouble breaking "bad habits"?

Are you very competitive/ do you compare

yourself with others a lot?

Are you well organized?

Do you check and re-check the alarm clock to

make sure it is set at night?

Are you good at planning? Do you get upset easily

if plans change?

Issues between 1am – 3am??

Depending on your answers to these questions, you will see which elements and meridians are out of balance. Then, when you are ready to sting your extremities, you will have some new ideas of which acupuncture pathways might help you the most. I am always available for consultations to help you decide where to sting and a good treatment plan.

My email address is: forever_amber_rose@yahoo.com

My FB address is: https://www.facebook.com/AmberRoseForever

CHAPTER 3

MANIFESTATIONS OF THE WOOD ELEMENT

You have chosen to work on the wood element. The wood element has two pathways associated with it, the gall bladder and the liver. This section is designed to give you the information you need to decide if one of those pathways is more important for you than the other.

Please circle or underline any characteristics or symptoms that relate to you on the gall bladder pathway and then on the liver pathway. When you are done, select the pathway you want to begin with. Turn to the treatment plan for that pathway and follow the directions. When you are ready, you can switch to the other pathway.

If you cannot decide which pathway you want to start with, it is OK to work on both pathways simultaneously. Remember to keep good, clear records of what you do. That way, if you have good results you can duplicate your experience. Also, good records will enable us to gather more information to help others in the future.

After you have worked on the wood element for a while, you may want to consider starting on another element. You can always come back to the wood pathways when you need to.

You may want to pay extra special attention to the wood element in the season associated with it, spring, and also when you notice symptoms that go with the wood element.

THE GALL BLADDER

Circle or underline any item(s) on this page that you feel relate to you:

POSITIVE QUALITIES:
When the pathway is in balance, the person makes good decisions; has good judgment, good vision, good sense of direction; concerned with fairness and justice; ability to assert self; flexible; good coordination; good organizational skills; wants to grow, able to move

forward and see clearly; may be very creative, such as artists, dancers, or musicians.

PHYSICAL CONDITIONS (ESPECIALLY IN CHILDHOOD) THAT MAY CAUSE OR SIGNAL AN IMBALANCE IN THE GALLBLADDER:

When this pathway is out of balance, the person may have these physical problems: issues with the gall bladder; eye problems; problems of ligaments and tendons; i.e., MS, myofacial pain, fibromyalgia, bursitis, arthritis, frozen joints (shoulders, elbows, knees or especially hip); coordination problems; one-sided complaints (especially one-sided headaches), pains that migrate and move around; alcohol or drug-related problems; low energy; many scars (especially large scars—any time there is a scar, the gall bladder has to make a decision on how to heal the person—how soon someone gets well from any illness or injury depends on the gall bladder); dry or brittle nails, nail biting; allergies; addictions; headaches due to anger; buzzing in the ears; migrating pains; dry, brittle nails; difficulty with any symptoms or issues between 11 p.m. and 3 a.m. (waking up or being more creative in those hours); likes or dislikes wind, spring, sour foods, the color green. The person shouts a lot or has a very quiet voice that sounds "breathy."

EMOTIONAL/SPIRITUAL IMBALANCES OF THE GALLBLADDER:

When this pathway is out of balance the person may have the following emotional/spiritual problems: difficulty making decisions; confusion or "wishy-washiness"; can't finish projects; easily intimidated, non-assertive, shy, weak, procrastination, lack of direction, no growth (artists who feel blocked and can't grow, "writers' block"); frustration, anger, impatience; very judgmental, rigid, punishing and judging others; sergeant type of a person with inconstancy, "hard on the outside and soft on the inside"; pushy; negative; no "give"; blind to reality around him/her; very in tune to fairness—go crazy if things are not fair; has trouble with hierarchy; agitation, "can't sit still," fighting in school, rebellious in childhood, can't stand anything out of order; splits—left/right, top/bottom—feels pulled apart, identity issues; pays either a great deal of attention to details or no attention at all; difficulty with timing or feeling that there is not enough time; career issues; soft voice but angry inside; screams a lot; depression—due to anger held in or frustration at lack of growth.

THE LIVER

Circle or underline any item(s) on this page that you feel relate to you: POSITIVE QUALITIES:

When this pathway is in balance, the person excels in planning and organization, plans every activity for survival; guards the body from outside insults and inside toxicities; plans for the future (visual clarity and order); the architect who sees the big picture and makes plans and blueprints, and has goals; a person who has direction, knows where he's going and knows his place in life; sense of serenity, feels hopeful, wants to grow, able to break habits, can move forward, has hindsight, foresight, and insight; can put things in perspective; plans for growth and birth; stands tall against the wind, well-rooted; very hopeful; good muscle power to push through things.

PHYSICAL CONDITIONS (ESPECIALLY IN CHILDHOOD) THAT MAY CAUSE OR SIGNAL AN IMBALANCE IN THE LIVER :

When this pathway is out of balance, the person may have these physical problems: liver problems, hepatitis, jaundice, allergies, migraine headaches or headaches that feel like a tight band around the head; headaches when anger is stuck in the head; addictions to drugs or alcohol; problems with the immune system; problems with tendons and ligaments; MS, fibromyalgia, joint problems, rheumatic pains, pains that move around; eye problems (especially blurred vision); gynecological problems with blood flow; inability to recuperate, trouble bouncing back from illness; trouble getting up and sitting down; issues of glycolysis; problems with nails/nail biting; fatigue, achy limbs, difficulty with the wind; symptoms or issues between 1 a.m. and 3 a.m. (especially when waking then, or more creative then); likes or dislikes spring, sour food, the color green, and the wind. The person shouts a lot or has a very quiet, "breathy" voice.

41

EMOTIONAL/SPIRITUAL IMBALANCES OF THE LIVER:

When this pathway is out of balance the person may have the following emotional/spiritual problems: trouble making plans, trouble when plans change, no clear goals, "has no future," deep sense of hopelessness, or jumping into the future, not living in the present; easily blown over, not rooted, trouble breaking habits, impatient, frustrated; over-planning, checks and rechecks to see if alarm is set, if stove is off, if door is locked; green with envy, very competitive, makes comparisons between self and others (comparing one's inside to someone else's outside), walking around aimlessly and "feeling lost"; people who have never really grown up, stuck in anger, really intense; career issues (has many different careers or "doesn't know what they want to be when they grow up"); very soft voice but angry inside, or screams a lot; angry at self (may cause auto-immune diseases), self-criticism; not being able to see the forest for the trees, losing sight of your goals, operating in the dark, can't see where you are going and therefore you are in the dark, easily irritated, angry, "don't bother me"; lack of focus, sitting on anger, sour grapes, sourpuss, relationships "go sour," addictive personality, depression when you can't see a future, holding anger in or feeling like you're not growing.

CHAPTER 4

MANIFESTATIONS OF THE FIRE ELEMENT

You have chosen to work on the fire element. The fire element has four pathways associated with it: the heart, the small intestine, the heart protector (pericardium), and the three heater. This section is designed to give you the information you need to decide if one of those pathways is more important for you than the others.

Please circle or underline any characteristics or symptoms that relate to you on each of the four pathways. When you are done, select the pathway you want to begin with. Turn to the treatment plan for that pathway and follow the directions.

When you are ready, you can begin to work on the other pathways. If you cannot decide which pathway you want to start with, it is OK to work on all of them simultaneously. But you must remember to keep good, clear records of what you do. That way, if you have good results you can duplicate your experience. Also, good records will enable us to gather more information to help others in the future.

After you have worked on the fire element for a while, you may want to choose another element to start on. You can always come back to the fire element when you need to.

You may want to pay extra special attention to the fire element during the season that is associated with it, summer, and when you are having symptoms that are related to it.

THE HEART: THE SUPREME CONTROLLER

Circle or underline any item(s) on this page that you feel relate to you:

POSITIVE QUALITIES:
When this pathway is in balance, the person has integrity; is very responsible for coordinating the whole, like the conductor of an orchestra; treats each person as important; has a quality of

selflessness and unconditional love; is very insightful and wise; has a need to communicate, care, and give.

PHYSICAL CONDITIONS (ESPECIALLY IN CHILDHOOD) THAT MAY CAUSE OR SIGNAL AN IMBALANCE IN THE HEART :

When this pathway is out of balance, the person may have these physical problems: high fevers, especially scarlet fever, rheumatic fever, measles; heart murmurs and congenital heart and circulation problems; a history of electric shock treatments, electrical accidents, shocks, being struck by lightning; pain down the arm and up the throat; a history of sexual abuse, fibromyalgia, being in a fire; feeling better or worse between 11 a.m. and l p.m.; likes or dislikes the bitter taste, fires, the color red, summer, and heat. The sound of the voice is either happy (with lots of laughter) or is flat (lack of laugh).

EMOTIONAL/SPIRITUAL IMBALANCES OF THE HEART:

When this pathway is out of balance, the person may have the following emotional/spiritual problems: wants to be the center of attention; feels overwhelmed with too much responsibility; may treat a person like a thing; likes to be in control or has an issue with control, may feel out of control (a feeling of panic); defensive, may experience themselves as a failure, feels betrayed; coldness on every level, (physical, emotional, or spiritual); keeps busy; denial of the whole, lack of joy: "I feel dead or empty"; everything looks OK on the outside, but everything is mechanical on the inside; "I feel like my heart is encased in cement," or "I feel drained of life"; if this pathway is out of balance, you may get symptoms associated with the other elements and other pathways—if you see yourself in all of the elements, and can't decide which element is your primary issue, it may be the heart.

THE SMALL INTESTINE

Circle or underline any item(s) on this page that you feel relate to you:

POSITIVE QUALITIES:

When this pathway is in balance, the person is concerned with separating the pure from the impure, sends the pure food to the spleen for distribution and the garbage to the colon for elimination; ability to sort out all of life's experiences; ability to transform suffering into joy (an alchemist); to see clearly, to know the difference between self and others, to know what belongs where, "I know what's best and what's destructive to me."

PHYSICAL CONDITIONS (ESPECIALLY IN CHILDHOOD) THAT MAY CAUSE OR SIGNAL AN IMBALANCE IN THE SMALL INTESTINE :

When this pathway is out of balance, the person may have these physical problems: high fevers, measles; fibromyalgia; ear problems; small intestine blockage, digestive problems, or boils; being in a fire; feels better or worse between l:00 p.m. and 3:00 p.m.; likes or dislikes the color red, heat, summer, and the bitter taste. The person's voice will have a lot of laughter in it or may be flat with no joy at all.

EMOTIONAL/SPIRITUAL IMBALANCES OF THE SMALL INTESTINE:

When this pathway is out of balance, the person may have the following emotional/spiritual problems: feeling "spacey" or confused, can't sort things out, life is cluttered (like an old Victorian house), too many options and the person doesn't know what to do, "maybe I'll do this, no . . . maybe I'll do that . . . no, I think I'll do that"; absent-minded professor; wanting to run away from problems when they don't know what to do; joyless, feeling polluted, feeling their energy is clogged up; problems of separation, sorting and choosing poorly, leaving you in situations or relationships where you may get hurt or stay with people who are not good for you.

THE HEART PROTECTOR / PERICARDIUM

Circle or underline any item(s) on this page that you feel relate to you:

POSITIVE QUALITIES:

When this pathway is in balance, the heart is well protected from the bumps and bruises of life, the person doesn't get her feelings hurt easily (there is good protection); he carries the essence of the heart out to others; good sexual function; good circulatory function; the "gatekeeper of the castle moat," knows when to open and close the drawbridge and let people in and out, knows how to be intimate, doesn't feel vulnerable, and feels well protected.

PHYSICAL CONDITIONS (ESPECIALLY IN CHILDHOOD) THAT MAY CAUSE OR SIGNAL AN IMBALANCE IN THE HEART PROTECTOR :

When this pathway is out of balance, the person may have the following physical conditions: high fevers, especially rheumatic fever, scarlet fever, measles; heart problems, sexual problems, sexual abuse, rapes; fibromyalgia; shoulders tend to slump forward; circulation problems, interruption in cardiac rhythm, angina, palpitations, cold hands and cold feet; problems between 7:00 p.m. and 9:00 p.m.; likes or dislikes the color red, summer, heat, fires, and the bitter taste. The person's voice is either happy and filled with laughter or flat (lack of joy).

EMOTIONAL/SPIRITUAL IMBALANCES OF THE HEART PROTECTOR:

When this pathway is out of balance, the person may experience the following emotional/spiritual problems: issues of trust, fear of being hurt/rejected, feeling unloved, relationship issues, wanting unconditional love, feeling unprotected and vulnerable, easily hurt, wearing your heart on your shirtsleeve, not feeling safe, loss of memory to protect oneself, lack of intimacy or craving intimacy, putting walls up to protect oneself, self-deception to protect oneself, issues of chemistry in a relationship, heartbreak in a relationship, sexual issues (impotence, frigidity); fear of being cold; depression due to feeling unloved or that you've displeased someone.

THE "THREE HEATER"

Circle or underline any item(s) on this page that you feel relate to you:

POSITIVE QUALITIES:

When this pathway is in balance, the person may be good at balance and harmony, enjoys being the peacemaker; works to create a perfect environment, a networker, good at receiving and transmitting information (a TV or radio announcer), good conversationalist, good debater; perfect hostess, loves to touch/ hug and be touched/hugged, enjoys groups, keeps the family in touch, sends birthday cards etc., and brings warmth to situations.

PHYSICAL CONDITIONS (ESPECIALLY IN CHILDHOOD) THAT MAY CAUSE OR SIGNAL AN IMBALANCE IN THE THREE HEATER:

When this pathway is out of balance, the person may experience the following physical problems: high fevers, measles, feeling too hot or too cold (the thermostat within the body is out of balance), cold hands and cold feet; fibromyalgia; affected by the environment (a butcher going in and out of the freezer; a person going in and out of a hot tub, sauna, using an electric blanket, etc.); feels hot and cold, has fear of cold and wears many layers of clothing or feels warm and wears less clothing then most people on a cold day, breathing problems due to not enough heat in the lungs; withdraws heat, warmth from organs (like pelvis—difficulty conceiving); being in a fire, speech impediments or stuttering, hearing problems, problems between 9 p.m. and 11 p.m.; likes or dislikes bitter taste, the color red, summer, and heat. The person has a joyful and laughing voice or one that is flat with no joy.

EMOTIONAL/SPIRITUAL IMBALANCES OF THE THREE HEATER:

When this pathway is out of balance, the person may experience the following emotional/spiritual problems: having to be the peacemaker in your family and not liking it; not feeling loved ("I have all these friends—but I don't feel loved"), constantly trying to connect to be loved, inability to make social contacts, can't discriminate between social and intimate

47

contacts, feeling that you're nice to them one day and they think you are their best friend), or they can't reach out ("I don't know anybody"), they always have some excuse for not reaching out or they hide in their one relationship and have trouble reaching out from it; withdrawing love from others, depression due to feeling unloved or that you've displeased someone; pulling back one's love or needing to give out a lot of warmth and love; may have difficulty with groups or public speaking, stuttering, speech impediments.

CHAPTER 5

MANIFESTATIONS OF THE EARTH ELEMENT

You have chosen to work on the earth element. The earth element has two pathways associated with it, the stomach and the spleen. This section is designed to give you the information you need to decide if one of those pathways is more important for you than the other.

Please circle or underline any characteristics or symptoms that relate to you on the stomach pathway and then on the spleen pathway. When you are done, select the pathway you want to begin with. Turn to the treatment plan for that pathway and follow the directions. When you are ready, you can work on the other pathway.

If you cannot decide which pathway you want to start with, it is OK to work on both pathways simultaneously. Remember to keep good, clear records of what you do. That way, if you have good results you can duplicate your experience. Also, good records will enable us to gather more information to help others in the future.

After you have worked on the earth element for a while, you may want to choose another element to work on. You can always come back to the earth element whenever you need to.

You may want to pay extra special attention to the earth element in the season associated with it, late summer, or when you are having symptoms related to the earth element.

THE STOMACH

Circle or underline any item(s) on this page that you feel relate to you:

POSITIVE QUALITIES:

When this pathway is in balance, the person has a good digestive system, receives and provides nourishment to the body; is very nurturing and empathetic; integrates and processes well; reliable, steady, centered.

PHYSICAL CONDITIONS (ESPECIALLY IN CHILDHOOD) THAT MAY CAUSE OR SIGNAL AN IMBALANCE IN THE STOMACH:

When this pathway is out of balance, the person may experience the following physical problems: digestion problems, belching, burping, anorexia, bulimia, cramps, leg pains, muscle problems, MS, chronic fatigue syndrome; nausea, vomiting; diabetes, hypoglycemia, headaches due to hypoglycemia; loves sweets, needing to chew gum or have something sweet in one's mouth; overweight, unusual distribution of weight, lumps, difficult pregnancies, miscarriages; hiatal hernia; problems between 7:00 a.m.—9:00 a.m., "a morning person" or "definitely not a morning person"; likes or dislikes humidity, late summer, and the colors yellow, orange, and brown. The sound of the voice has either a singing quality to it or it is monotone.

EMOTIONAL/SPIRITUAL IMBALANCES OF THE STOMACH:

When this pathway is out of balance, the person may experience the following emotional/spiritual problems: craving sympathy, empathy, very needy and clingy, or taking care of everyone else but not asking for help yourself; lack of centeredness, never feeling satisfied, "poor me," craving to be understood or feeling misunderstood, "hungry or starved" for love or sex (pawing), caretaker, needing to be needed, depression due to feeling needy and starving, and having trouble with "the empty nest syndrome."

THE SPLEEN

Circle or underline any item(s) on this page that you feel relate to you:

POSITIVE QUALITIES:

When this pathway is in balance, the person has good energy, maintains good blood sugar levels, lymphatic system in good shape, the body has the ability to protect itself; a sense of fulfillment with life, enjoys bringing children into the world.

PHYSICAL CONDITIONS (ESPECIALLY IN CHILDHOOD) THAT MAY CAUSE OR SIGNAL AN IMBALANCE IN THE SPLEEN:

When this pathway is out of balance, the person may experience the following physical problems: muscle problems, MS, feeling sluggish, chronic tiredness, chronic fatigue syndrome, listlessness, feels unable to pick up their hand, "my legs can't carry me where I want to go," heaviness, spinning, dizziness, craves or dislikes sweets, diabetes, hypoglycemia and blood sugar issues, including headaches; long term chronic illness that doesn't seem to have much cause; overweight and unusual distribution of weight, leg pain, a sagging feeling; trouble at 9 a.m. — 11 a.m. or loves 9 a.m. — 11 a.m.; likes or dislikes humidity, late summer, and the colors yellow, orange, and brown. The person's voice is either singing or monotone.

EMOTIONAL/SPIRITUAL IMBALANCES OF THE SPLEEN:

When this pathway is out of balance, the person may experience the following emotional/spiritual problems: inability to cope with little daily things, inability to stop obsessiveness, belaboring issues, paying attention to petty details; nightmares, especially with aspect of things spinning (going in circles); not carrying things to fruition, can't carry fetus to full term; giving too much, not taking care of oneself, smothering, overly sweet; paying too much attention to the body, lots of symptoms and no one can find a cause; very needy, almost draining, holding onto one's children, lack of peacefulness, depression due to fatigue or feeling needy (starving, tired).

CHAPTER 6

MANIFESTATIONS OF THE METAL ELEMENT

You have chosen to work on the metal element. The metal element has two pathways associated with it, the lung and the colon. This section is designed to give you the information you need to decide if one of those pathways is more important for you than the other.

Please circle or underline any characteristics or symptoms that relate to you on the lung pathway and then on the colon pathway. When you are done, select the pathway you want to begin with. Turn to the treatment plan for that pathway and follow the directions. When you are ready, you can start on the other pathway.

If you cannot decide which pathway you want to start with, it is OK to work on both pathways simultaneously. Remember to keep good, clear records of what you do. That way, if you have good results you can duplicate your experience. Also, good records will enable us to gather more information to help others in the future.

After you have worked on this element for a while you might want to consider choosing another element to start on. You can always come back to the metal element when you need to.

You may want to pay extra special attention to the metal element in the season associated with it, the autumn, or when you are having symptoms related to the metal element.

THE LUNGS

Circle or underline any item(s) on this page that you feel relate to you:

POSITIVE QUALITIES:

When this pathway is in balance, the person feels very connected to the universe and to God, really into quality, brilliance, self-worth; easily inspired and gives inspiration to others; ability to receive and welcome;

good relations with father; a sense of rhythmic order of life, aware of what is precious in life; "he is my rock of Gibraltar," rock-like structure, steadiness; good with finances; able to give and receive; never feels alone.

PHYSICAL CONDITIONS (ESPECIALLY IN CHILDHOOD) THAT MAY CAUSE OR SIGNAL AN IMBALANCE IN THE LUNGS :

When this pathway is out of balance, the person may experience the following physical problems: lung problems, pleurisy, pneumonia, bronchitis, asthma, allergies, skin problems (the skin is the third lung), coughs, sore throats, mononucleosis; leukemia, environmental illness; excess mucus, dairy allergies, craving spicy foods or has trouble with them; smokers; congestion headaches; trouble sleeping between 3 a.m. and 5 a.m.; likes or dislikes dryness, the color white, and autumn; wears a lot of metal jewelry or can't wear any. The sound of the person's voice is sad and weepy.

EMOTIONAL/SPIRITUAL IMBALANCES OF THE LUNG:

When this pathway is out of balance, the person may experience the following emotional/spiritual problems: difficulty receiving love and compliments, feeling cut off, a loner, lack of self-worth, feeling inadequate; difficult relationship with guru, looking for what his own father never gave him, looking to fill emptiness or a void, lonely, wanting to be special, feeling unappreciated, feeling unworthy, guilty; trouble with money issues; negativity, depression, "going manic," soaring to the heights and plunging to the depths; helped by meditation; smokers who feel as if their cigarettes are like a companion ("maybe now that I'm in this relationship I'll be able to give up smoking"), grief, loss, sadness, the pain of giving someone something and they don't or can't receive it; likes vacations in the mountains; fear of being alone; speech difficulties, a weak voice or trouble getting the words out, or a "know-it-all" who feels much superior to everyone else; wears excess jewelry.

THE COLON (LARGE INTESTINE)

Circle or underline any item(s) on this page that you feel relate to you:

53

POSITIVE QUALITIES:

When this pathway is in balance, the person lets go easily and without effort, faith that quality and abundance are available, able to detach when necessary; able to grieve and then let go; feels special and unique; large intestine moves well; neat and clean; loves the mountains, feels connected to the universe, goes for quality; knows what to retain and what to let go.

PHYSICAL CONDITIONS (ESPECIALLY IN CHILDHOOD) THAT MAY CAUSE OR SIGNAL AN IMBALANCE IN THE COLON:

When this pathway is out of balance, the person may experience the following physical problems: severe diarrhea or constipation, dysentery, spastic colon; hernias; mononucleosis; leukemia, environmental illness; excess mucus, dairy allergies, difficulties with the nose or sinuses and sense of smell; headaches (when the mind is clogged "like a NYC garbage strike inside the body"); fatigue; eye problems; scanty menstruation; poor circulation headaches due to being stuck in negativity; wakes between 5 a.m. and 7 a.m.; likes or dislikes autumn, spicy food, and the color white. The person's voice sounds sad and weepy.

EMOTIONAL/SPIRITUAL IMBALANCES OF THE COLON:

When this pathway is out of balance, the person may experience the following emotional/spiritual problems: unforgiving, obstinate ("that old battle ax"), stuck, stubborn; a harsh or twisted person, negative thinkers, complainers; sense of futility or alienation, despair; low self-esteem, think they are shit; live in the past (the past is still alive in them).

CHAPTER 7

MANIFESTATIONS OF THE WATER ELEMENT

You have chosen to work on the water element. The water element has two pathways associated with it, the bladder and the kidney. This section is designed to give you the information you need to decide if one of those pathways is more important for you than the other.

Please circle or underline any characteristics or symptoms that relate to you on the bladder pathway and then on the kidney pathway. When you are done, select the pathway you want to begin with. Turn to the treatment plan for that pathway and follow the directions. When you are ready, you can work on the other pathway.

If you cannot decide which pathway you want to start with, it is OK to work on both pathways simultaneously. Remember to keep good, clear records of what you do. That way, if you have good results you can duplicate your experience. Also, good records will enable us to gather more information to help others in the future.

After you have worked on the water element for a while, you may feel ready to move onto another element. Feel free to do this. You can always come back to the water element when you need it.

You may want to pay extra special attention to the water element in the season associated with it, winter, or when you are having symptoms related to the water element.

THE BLADDER

Circle or underline any item(s) on this page that you feel relate to you:

POSITIVE QUALITIES:

When this pathway is in balance, the person has the ability to store fluids including urine and thus maintain adequate reserves for emergencies, elasticity, courage, willpower; ability to stretch to the limits, flexible.

PHYSICAL CONDITIONS (ESPECIALLY IN CHILDHOOD) THAT MAY CAUSE OR SIGNAL AN IMBALANCE IN THE BLADDER:

When this pathway is out of balance, the person may experience the following physical problems: feeling tired (burnt out, burning your candle at both ends), feeling a tiredness as if someone has just pulled the plug (often between 3 p.m. and 5 p.m.); "my batteries are low"; environmental illness; lack of flexibility; headaches due to fear, frozen shoulders (frozen with fear); bladder problems; excess fluid (edema) swelling or dehydration; dislikes or likes cold weather, rain, salty foods, the colors blue and black; the person's voice sounds like a groan.

EMOTIONAL/SPIRITUAL IMBALANCES OF THE BLADDER:

When this pathway is out of balance, the person may experience the following emotional/spiritual problems: fear, or lack of fear (Evel Knievel), panic, terror, feeling overwhelmed, "I don't have anything left to give"; hibernates (isolates due to fear), afraid to experience ones emotions; needing to relax and replenish, wants a vacation by the water or to a cold climate; feeling depleted due to a sudden shock; when the fear is so great it's hard to have a relationship, frozen or paralyzed with fear, phobias, living on the edge, taking on the hardest projects and pushing oneself to the limits.

THE KIDNEYS

Circle or underline any item(s) on this page that you feel relate to you:

POSITIVE QUALITIES:

When this pathway is in balance, the person may be very energetic; clever, powerful, courageous, peaceful, ambitious, have strong willpower; "goes with the flow"; an inner drive from deep within.

PHYSICAL CONDITIONS (ESPECIALLY IN CHILDHOOD) THAT MAY CAUSE OR SIGNAL AN IMBALANCE IN THE KIDNEY:

When this pathway is out of balance, the person may experience the following physical problems: kidney problems, kidney stones, high fevers that burn up the fluids in the body, e.g., measles; edema (swelling due to too much fluid in the body), or dehydration, urinary problems, nephritis; issues with perspiration, and night sweats; dry eyes or dryness in the body; low back and/or knee pain; joint problems; shortness of breath, listlessness or fatigue; environmental illness; cold limbs; darkish face (especially dark circles around the eyes); headaches due to fear, birth defects or mental retardation; chronic ear aches or deafness; premature white or gray hair, baldness, bone problems, tooth problems; feels better or has problems that are more severe in winter or between 5 p.m. and 7 p.m.; likes or dislikes the colors blue/black and salty foods. The person's voice sounds like a groan.

EMOTIONAL/SPIRITUAL IMBALANCES OF THE KIDNEY:

When this pathway is out of balance, the person may experience the following emotional/spiritual problems: defects in will power, i.e., addictions, no will to stop smoking or drinking, no ambition; stuck because of fear, terror, or panic; giving up due to fear of life, "I just can't do it!," and very deep fears, paranoia or everything becomes the enemy (environmental illness, chemical sensitivity), or a total lack of fear (daredevil).

CHAPTER 8

INTRODUCTION TO TREATMENT PLANS

The following treatment plans suggest a number of approaches to selecting sting locations. Now that you have chosen the primary element(s) in which you want to work, these plans will assist you in preparing for a treatment session. According to the Chinese understanding of the meridians, each pathway contains specific points. Each meridian, for example, contains a point representing each element, so that whether the pathway is wood or fire, it will contain a point for all five elements. The element point which is the same as the pathway is a special point called the home element point. Each meridian also contains a series of special points, such as a source point, entry/exit points, a horary point, a junction point (luo), tonification, and sedation points. Some pathways also include points known as Windows of the Sky and Spirit points. These points can serve dual purposes on some meridians.

The suggested treatment plans incorporate classical acupuncture knowledge with my experience in the application of bees to this oriental system of healing. You may want to begin with a few stings (after test stings) on one pathway; this gives the body a clear instruction, and avoids confusion by trying to do too many things at the same time. This is in accordance with "The Law of Least Action"; while we are tempted to think that more is better, excessive instructions can send mixed messages and detract from simple clarity. As you develop an understanding of the five element system, you will learn to expand your sessions to include a greater number of points which exist in relationship to one another.

Once you've gone past the 2 - 3 month window, feel free to do your stings by combining acupuncture locations with "trigger points," "nerve meridians," scars, or any of the other suggestions in this book. Keep in mind doing test stings as you slowly creep down your extremities.

Some points are located in anatomical sites such that bee stings may be particularly uncomfortable. These points are ones which should be stung "with care." Some points may also itch or swell if you go there too early in your treatment. Therefore we 2 - 3 months before going to the extremities.

CHAPTER 9

TREATMENT PLAN - GALL BLADDER PATHWAY

Here is a possible treatment plan to work on the gallbladder (GB) pathway. This plan is immediately followed by locations and point names.

    I. If you want to strengthen the GB pathway, you can sting the tonification point (GB-43) or the source point (GB-40).

    2. If you want to connect the GB to its paired meridian, the liver (LV), sting yourself on the junction point (GB-37).

    3. You can enhance the effectiveness of your treatment by stinging the home element point (GB-41). This is best done as a horary treatment, which means a treatment on the home element point at the right time of day (11 p.m.—1 a.m.) and or in the right season (spring).

    4. If you are having symptoms between 11 p.m.—1 a.m., (i.e., having trouble going to sleep, or waking up at this time every night), then you may want to sting the entry point (GB-1), taking care because this point is close to the eye, and/or exit point (GB-41). Another time to consider stinging the entry/exit points is if you start to feel better and then you feel like you are going backwards. Your symptoms may go away or are alleviated, and then all of a sudden they return again. Instead of getting discouraged, try stinging the entry/exit points!

    5. Choose a specific point on the GB based on the name of the point. This is called treating by the spirit of the point. Look at the names of all the points on the GB pathway. Do any of the names jump out at you? What about Bright and Clear (GB 37)? That point is good for seeing things clearly. Do you have trouble with your eyes? Or are you confused? Bright and Clear may be the point for you. Or how about Neglected Muscles (GB 23); does that name bring up thoughts of muscles that have atrophied or are not being used? These are just two examples of some of the points that might speak to you.

6. Try combining any of the above recommendations. "BEE" creative. And remember to keep good records.

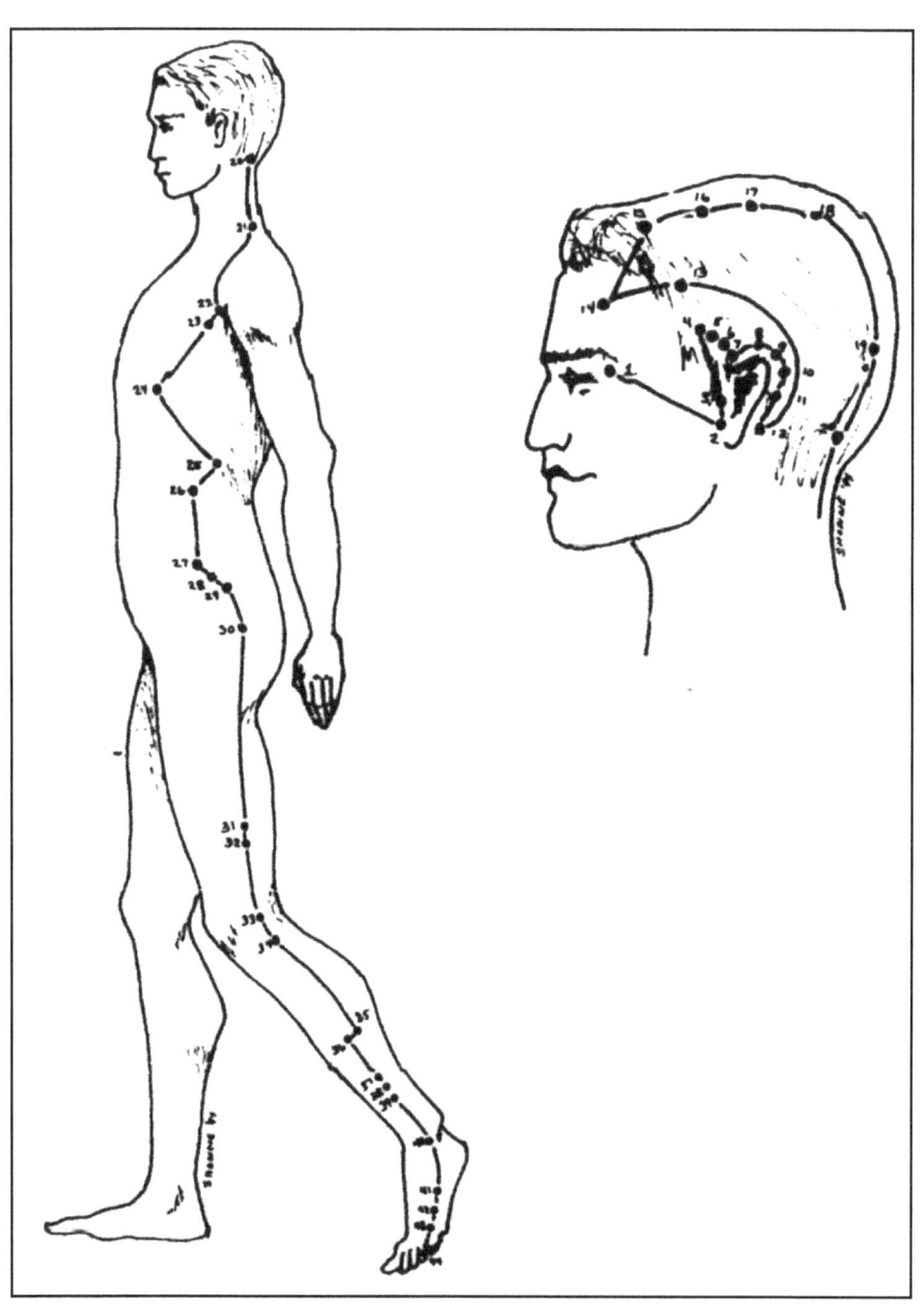

GALL BLADDER PATHWAY (GB)

GB-I   Orbit Bone (entry pt.)(Take care because this is close to the eye.)

GB-2   Hearing Assembly

GB-3   Upper Pass

GB-4   Forehead Fullness

GB-5   Suspended Skull

GB-6   Suspended Regulator

GB-7   Temporal Hairline Curve

GB-8   Valley Lead

GB-9   Heaven Rushing

GB-10 Floating White

GB-11 Head Porthole Yin

GB-12 Completion Bone

GB-13 Root Spirit

GB-14 Yang White

GB-15 Head Overlooking Tears

GB-16 Eye Window (This is not officially a Window to the Sky but it can be used that way for the whole wood element.)

GB-17 Upright Construction

GB-18 Receiving Spirit

GB-19 Brain Hollow

GB-20 Wind Pond (good pt. for muscles; first aid pt: poison)

GB-21 Shoulder Well

GB-22 Armpit Abyss

GB-23 Neglected Muscles

GB-24 Sun and Moon (A good pt. for someone who feels split, opposite polar feelings!)

GB-25 Capital Gate

GB-26 Girdle Vessel

GB-27 Fifth Pivot (good pt. for hip problems and balance)

GB-28 Binding Path (good pt. for hip problems and balance)

GB-29 Dwelling in the Bone (good pt. for hip problems and balance)

GB-30 Jumping Round (first aid pt: fractures and sprains)

GB-31 Wind Market

GB-32 Middle Ditch

GB-33 Knee Yang Joint

GB-34   Yang Mound Spring (earth pt. and assembling pt. of tendons, muscles; lack of coordination and paralysis, knee and ankle problems)

GB-35 Yang Crossing (good for chest, legs, feet, muscles)

GB-36 Outer Mound (a good pt. for intense dislike of wind)

GB-37   Bright and Clear (junction pt. and good pt. for eyes, paralysis, drug users, rigidity and spasm, coordinating muscles and tendons, and for those having trouble standing)

GB-38 Yang Support (fire and sedation pts.)

GB-39 Severed Bone (assembling pt. of marrow and meeting pt. of the bladder, gallbladder and stomach pathway; this pt. is good for bone marrow and cortisone production)

GB-40 Wilderness Mound (source pt., good spirit pt. for getting a perspective on your life; first aid pt: food poisoning, poison, lack of co-ordination, swelling and sighing)

GB-41 Foot Above Tears (This point is a wood, home element, exit and horary pts., 11 p.m.—1 a.m. This is a pt. related to getting above angry tears; a good pt. for rheumatism.)

GB-42 Earth Five-Fold

GB-43 Valiant Stream (water and tonification pts., good pt. for puffy face, too much or too little water; good to cool down anger and violence)

GB-44 Foot Hole Yin (metal pt., good pt. for inability to move arms and legs due to pain, inability to speak and bend knees, insomnia)

CHAPTER 10

TREATMENT PLAN - LIVER PATHWAY (LV)

Here is a possible treatment plan to work on the liver (LV) pathway. This plan is immediately followed by point names and locations.

l. If you want to strengthen the LV pathway, you can sting the tonification point (LV-8) or the source point (LV-3).

2. If you want to connect the LV to its paired meridian the gall bladder (GB), sting yourself on the junction point (LV-5). (See glossary for more information.)

3. You can enhance the effectiveness of your treatment by stinging the home element point (LV-1). This is best done as a horary treatment, which means a treatment on the home element point at the right time of day (1 a.m.— 3 a.m.) and/or in the right season (spring).

4. If you are having symptoms between 1 a.m.—3 a.m. (i.e., having trouble falling asleep then, or waking up at that time every night), then you may want to sting the entry point (LV-1) and/or the exit points (LV-13 and LV-14). Another reason to consider stinging the entry/exit points is if you start to feel better and then you feel like you are going backwards. Your symptoms may go away or are alleviated, and then all of a sudden they return again. Instead of getting discouraged, try stinging the entry/exit points!

5. Choose a specific point on the LV based on the name of the point. This is called treating by the spirit of the point. Look at the names of all the points on the LV pathway. Do any of the names jump out at you? What about Chapter Gate (LV-13)? This is all about starting a new chapter in your life. Does that sound like you? Or how about Gate of Hope (LV-14)? Are you feeling depressed or hopeless? Do you feel like nothing is ever going to change? These are just two examples of some of the points on the LV that might speak to you.

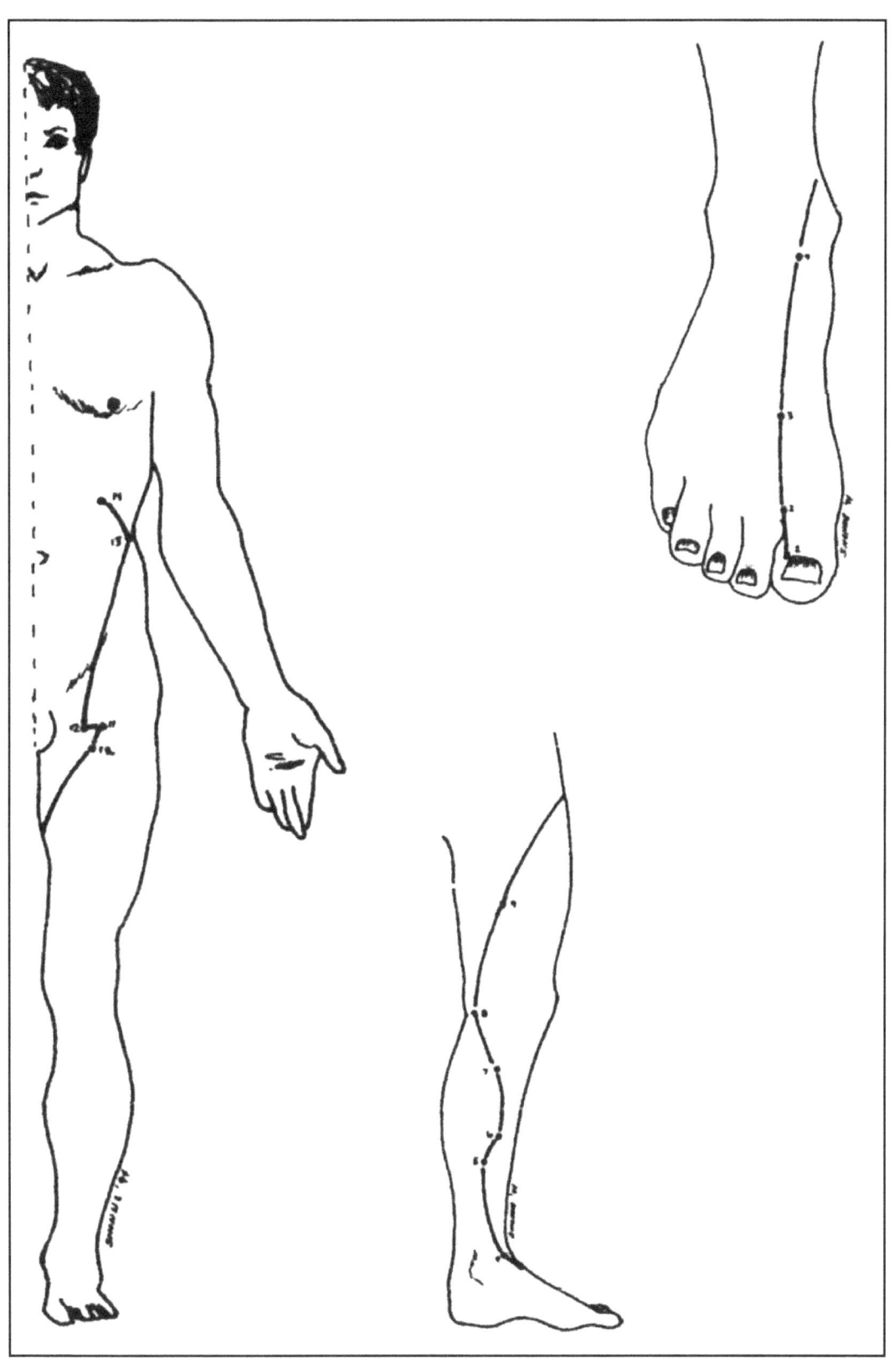

LIVER PATHWAY (LV)

LV-1 Great Esteem (wood, home element, entry, and horary pts., 1 a.m.—3 a.m.)

LV-2 Moving Between (fire and sedation pts., first aid pt: cramps, spasms)

LV-3 Happy Calm (earth and source pts., as well as a good pt. for getting toxins out of the body. This is a good pt. for allergies.)

LV-4 Middle Seal (metal pt. and a very good spiritual pt. for finding your identity; good pt. for cold legs and feet, muscle spasms, paralysis)

LV-5 Insect Ditch (junction pt. and a center of energy; this point is good if you feel like you are restless as if you have "ants in your pants"; a helpful point if you are unable to walk or stand; this is also good for cramps, abdominal pain, menstrual problems)

LV-6 Middle Capital (center of energy; first aid pt: cramps, spasms, and urine retention, also weakness and inability to stand, paralysis)

LV-7 Knee Joint (good for knee disorders)

LV-8 Spring at the Bend (water and tonification pts., a good pt. for urinary problems, fear, depression, anger, irritation, jealousy)

LV-9 Yin Wrapping

LV-10 Five Miles

LV-11 Yin Corner

LV-l2 Urgent Pulse

LV-13 Chapter Gate (exit pt., good for starting a new chapter in your life)

LV-14 Gate of Hope (exit pt. and good pt. for depression, despair, and feeling hopeless.)

67

CHAPTER 11

TREATMENT PLAN - HEART PATHWAY

Here is a possible treatment plan to work on the heart (H) pathway. This plan is immediately followed by point names and locations.

l. If you want to strengthen the H pathway, you can sting the tonification point (H-9) or the source point (H-7).

2. If you want to connect the H to its paired meridian the small intestine (SI), sting yourself on the junction point (H-5).

3. You can enhance the effectiveness of your treatment by stinging the home element point (H-8). This is best done as a horary treatment, which means a treat on the home element point at the right time of day (11 a.m.—1 p.m.) and/or in the right season (summer).

4. If you are having symptoms between 11 a.m.—1 p.m. (i.e., feeling tired or feeling depressed) you may want to sting the entry point (H-1) and/or the exit point (H-9). Another reason to consider stinging the entry/exit points is if you start to feel better and then you feel like you are going backwards. Your symptoms may go away or are alleviated, and then all of a sudden they return again. Instead of getting discouraged, try stinging the entry/exit points!

5. Choose a specific point on the H based on the name of the point. This is called treating by the spirit of the point. Look at the names of all the points on the H pathway. Do any of the names jump out at you? What about Spirit Path? (H-4) That is a point where you go to find your spiritual path. Or how about a point that will get to the heart of the matter, Penetrating Inside (H-5)? These are just two examples of some of the points on the H that might speak to you.

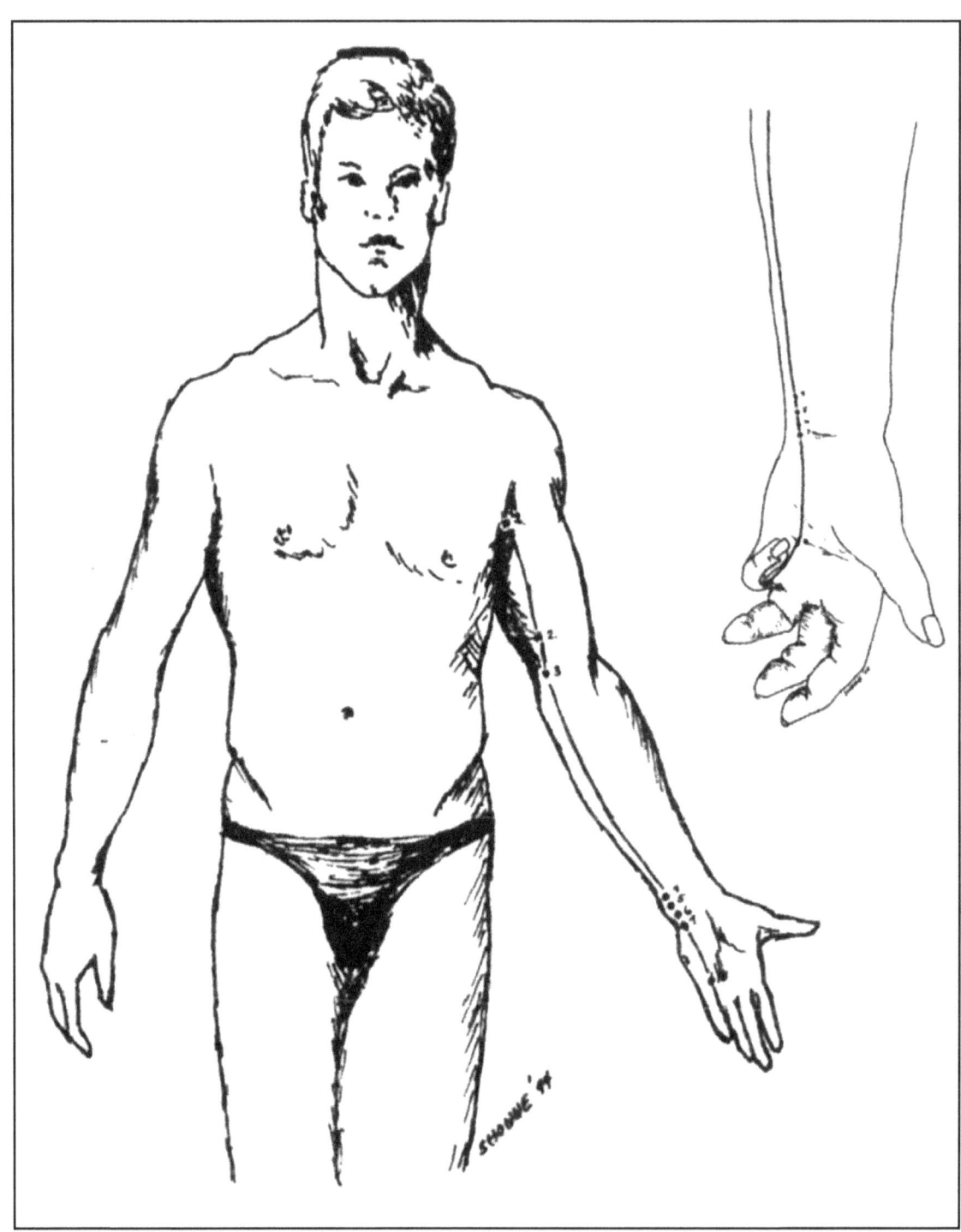

HEART PATHWAY (H)

H-1 Utmost Source (entry pt.)

H-2 Blue-Green Spirit

H-3 Lesser Sea (water pt.)

H-4 Spirit Path (metal pt.)

H-5 Penetrating Inside (junction pt.)

H-6 Yin Mound

H-7 Spirit Gate (earth, sedation, and source pts.)

H-8 Lesser Mansion (fire, home element, and horary pts., 11 a.m.—1 p.m.)

H-9 Lesser Surge (wood, tonification, and exit pts.)

CHAPTER 12

TREATMENT PLAN - SMALL INTESTINE

Here is a possible treatment plan to work on the small intestine (SI) pathway. This plan is immediately followed by point names and locations.

1. If you want to strengthen the SI pathway, you can sting the tonification point (SI-3) or the source point (SI-4).

2. If you want to connect the SI to its paired meridian the heart (H), sting yourself on the junction point (SI-7).

3. You can enhance the effectiveness of your treatment by stinging the home element point (SI-5). This is best done as a horary treatment, which means a treatment on the home element point at the right time of day (1 p.m.—3 p.m.) and/or in the right season (summer).

4. If you are having symptoms between 1 p.m.—3 p.m. (i.e., feeling tired or having trouble concentrating), then you may want to sting the entry point (SI- 1) and/or the exit point (SI-19). Another reason to consider stinging the entry/exit points is if you start to feel better and then you feel like you are going backwards. Your symptoms may go away or are alleviated, and then all of a sudden they return again. Instead of getting discouraged, try stinging the entry/exit points!

5. Choose a specific point on the SI based on the name of the point. This is called treating by the spirit of the point. Look at the names of all the points on the SI pathway. Do any of the names jump out at you? What about Nourishing the Old (SI- 6)? This point helps you let go of what you don't need from the past, but lets you treasure what was good. This is just one example of some of the points on the SI that might speak to you.

6. Also consider the possibility of stinging a Window of the Sky. The SI has two of them: (SI-16) and (SI-17). Windows of the Sky are traditionally done when you want to bring the body, mind, and spirit back into balance.

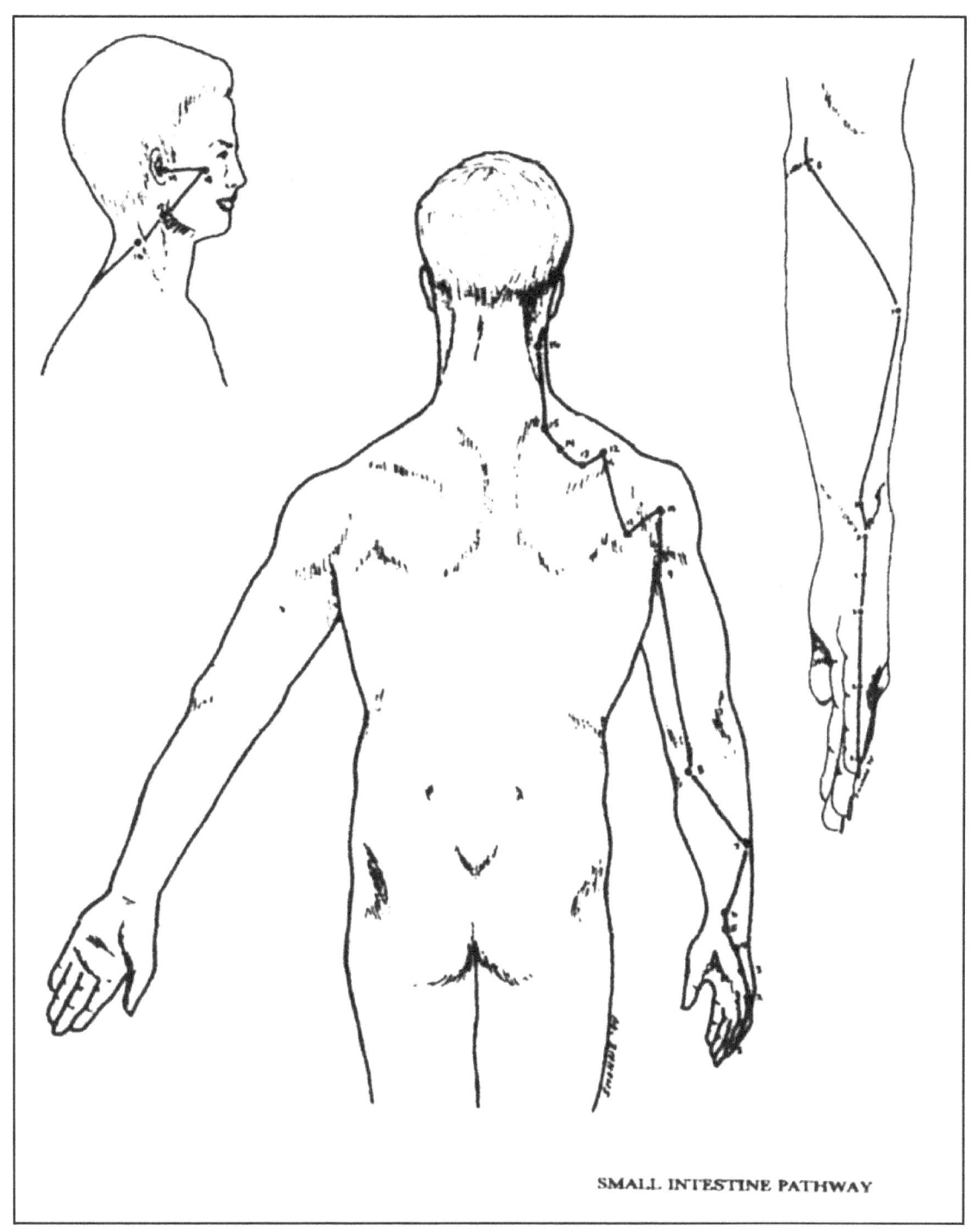

SMALL INTESTINE PATHWAY

SMALL INTESTINE PATHWAY (SI)

SI-1   Lesser Marsh (metal and entry pts.)

SI-2   Front Valley (water pt.)

SI-3   Back Ravine (wood and tonification pts.)

SI-4   Wrist Bone (source pt.)

SI-5   Yang Valley (fire, home element, and horary pts., 1 p.m.—3 p.m., good   pt. for tinnitus and Bell's Palsy)

SI-6   Nourishing the Old (a good spirit point for helping let go of things from the past that you don't need, yet treasure the good things)

SI-7   Branch to the Correct (junction pt.)

SI-8   Small Sea (earth and sedation pts.)

SI-9   True Shoulder

SI-10 Shoulder Blade

SI-11 Celestial Gathering

SI-12 Grasping the Wind

SI-13 Crooked Wall

SI-14 Outside the Shoulder Correspondence

SI-15 Middle of the Shoulder Correspondence

SI-16 Celestial Window (Window of the Sky)

SI-17 Heavenly Appearance (Window of the Sky)

SI-18 Cheek Bone-Hole (can use acupressure)

SI-19 Listening Palace (exit pt.)

CHAPTER 13

TREATMENT PLAN HEART PROTECTOR/PERICARDIUM PATHWAY

Here is a possible treatment plan to work on the heart protector (HP) pathway. This plan is immediately followed by point names and locations.

I. If you want to strengthen the HP pathway, you can sting the tonification point (HP-9) or the source point (HP-7).

2. If you want to connect the HP to its paired meridian the three heater (TH), sting yourself on the junction point (HP-6). (See glossary for more information.)

3. You can enhance the effectiveness of your treatment by stinging the horary point (HP-8) at the right time of day (7 p.m.—9 p.m.) and/or in the right season (summer).

4. If you are having symptoms between 7 p.m.—9 p.m. (i.e., feeling tired or feeling depressed) you may want to sting the entry point (HP-1 for men/HP-2 for women) and/or the exit point (HP-8). Another reason to consider stinging the entry/exit points is if you start to feel better and then you feel like you are going backwards. Your symptoms may go away or are alleviated, and then all of a sudden they return again. Instead of getting discouraged, try stinging the entry/exit points!

5. Choose a specific point on the HP based on the name of the point. This is called treating by the spirit of the point. Look at the names of all the points on the HP pathway. Do any of the names jump out at you? What about Palace of Weariness (HP-8)? That is a palace where you go to rejuvenate yourself. Or how about Inner Frontier Gate (HP-6)? This opens the gate to communicate with others on a more intimate level. These are just two examples of some of the points on the H that might speak to you.

6. You might want to consider stinging a Window of the Sky (HP-I for men and HP-2 for women). This will bring the body, mind, and spirit together.

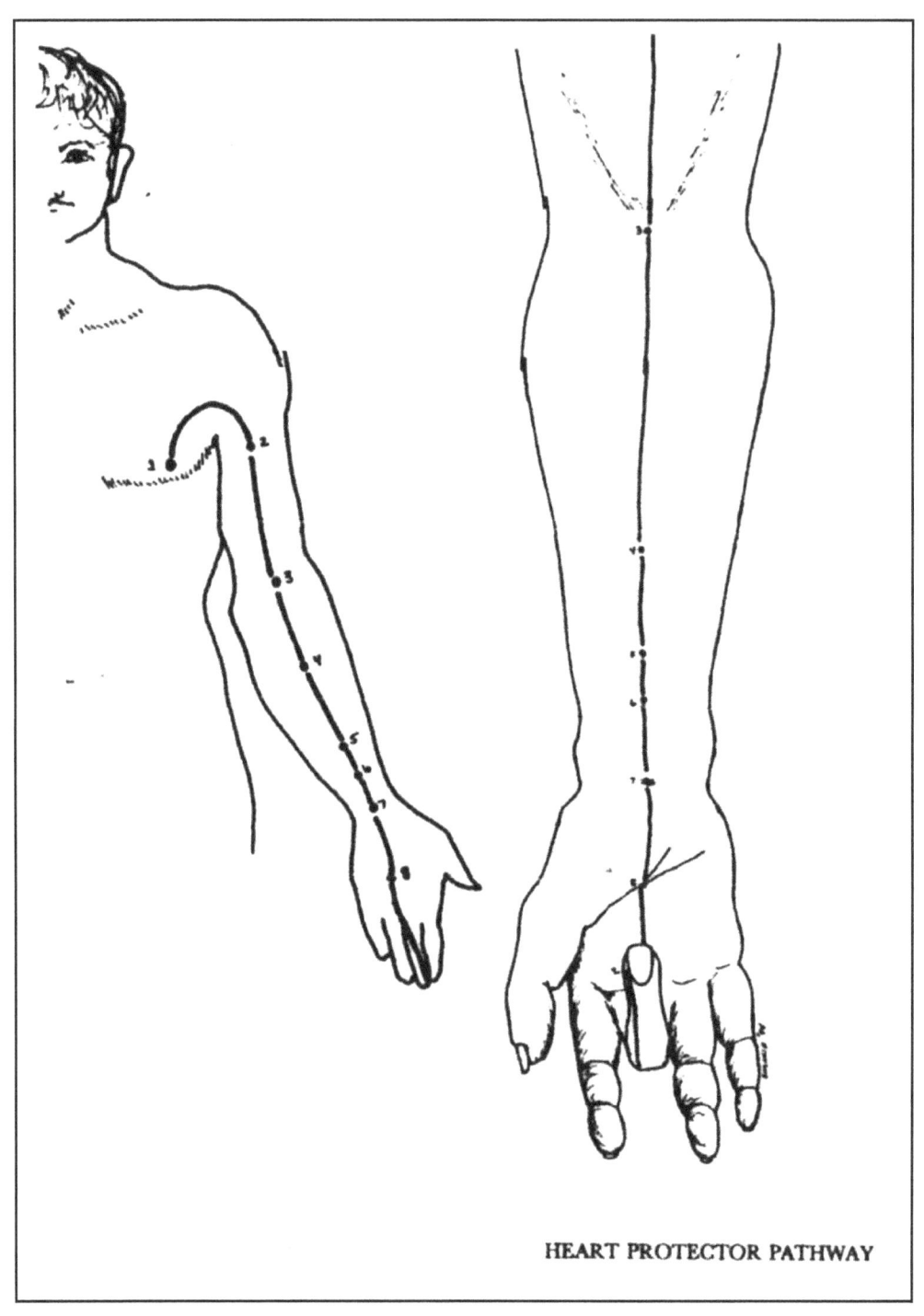

HEART PROTECTOR PATHWAY

HEART PROTECTOR PATHWAY (HP)

HP-1 Celestial Pool (entry pt. for men and Window of the Sky) - Forbidden in women

HP-2 Celestial Spring (entry pt. for women and Window of the Sky)

HP-3 Marsh at the Bend (water pt., a good pt. for someone who has a fear of water and of meeting people)

HP-4 Gate of Ch'i Reserve (a good pt. for a patient who feels that he or she has no energy and can't go on, an excellent pt. for a person who is suffering on the mental level)

HP-5 Intermediary Courier (metal pt., good pt. for grief in the heart, turning to God, a good pt. for food lying heavy in stomach)

HP-6 Inner Frontier Gate (junction pt., good point for anxiety and depression)

HP-7 Great Mound (earth, sedation and source pts. for fevers with much weariness, for people who are very sad; lack of stability and lack of control)

HP-8 Palace of Weariness (fire, home element, exit and horary pts., 7 p.m.—9 p.m., with this point closed, it is hard to have a successful marriage; lack of warmth, and lack of tolerance, asthma; a good point for those who are trying to be warm and loving, and yet feel they want to give up, and then become sad, miserable, or rigid)

HP-9 Central Hub (wood and tonification pts., first aid pt: anxiety and resuscitation, varicose veins, epilepsy)

CHAPTER 14

TREATMENT PLAN - THREE HEATER PATHWAY (TH)

Here is a possible treatment plan to work on the three heater (TH) pathway. This plan is immediately followed by point names and locations.

I. If you want to strengthen the TH pathway, you can sting the tonification point (TH-3) or the source point (TH-4).

2. If you want to connect the TH to its paired meridian the heart protector (HP), sting yourself on the junction point (TH-5).

3. You can enhance the effectiveness of your treatment by stinging the home element point (TH-6). This is best done as a horary treatment, which means a treatment on the home element point at the right time of day (9 p.m.—11 p.m.) and/or in the right season (summer).

4. If you are having symptoms between 9 p.m.—11 p.m. (i.e., having trouble falling asleep then, or feeling depressed), then you may want to sting the entry point (TH-1) and/or the exit point (TH-22). Another reason to consider stinging the entry/exit points is if you start to feel better and then you feel like you are going backwards. Your symptoms may go away or are alleviated, and then all of a sudden they return again. Instead of getting discouraged, try stinging the entry/exit points!

5. Choose a specific point on the TH based on the name of the point. This is called treating by the spirit of the point. Look at the names of all the points on the TH pathway. Do any of the names jump out? What about Pure Cold Abyss (TH-11)? Does that sound like you? Do you ever feel really cold and can't get warm? This is just one example of some of the points that might speak to you.

6. You also might want to consider doing a Window of the Sky (TH-16). This is a good point for bringing the body, mind, and spirit together. If you are seeking a breakthrough, this may be a good point for you. It is also located behind and just below the mastoid process of

the ear, so this is a good place to sting for balance, hearing problems, vision, and mental clarity.

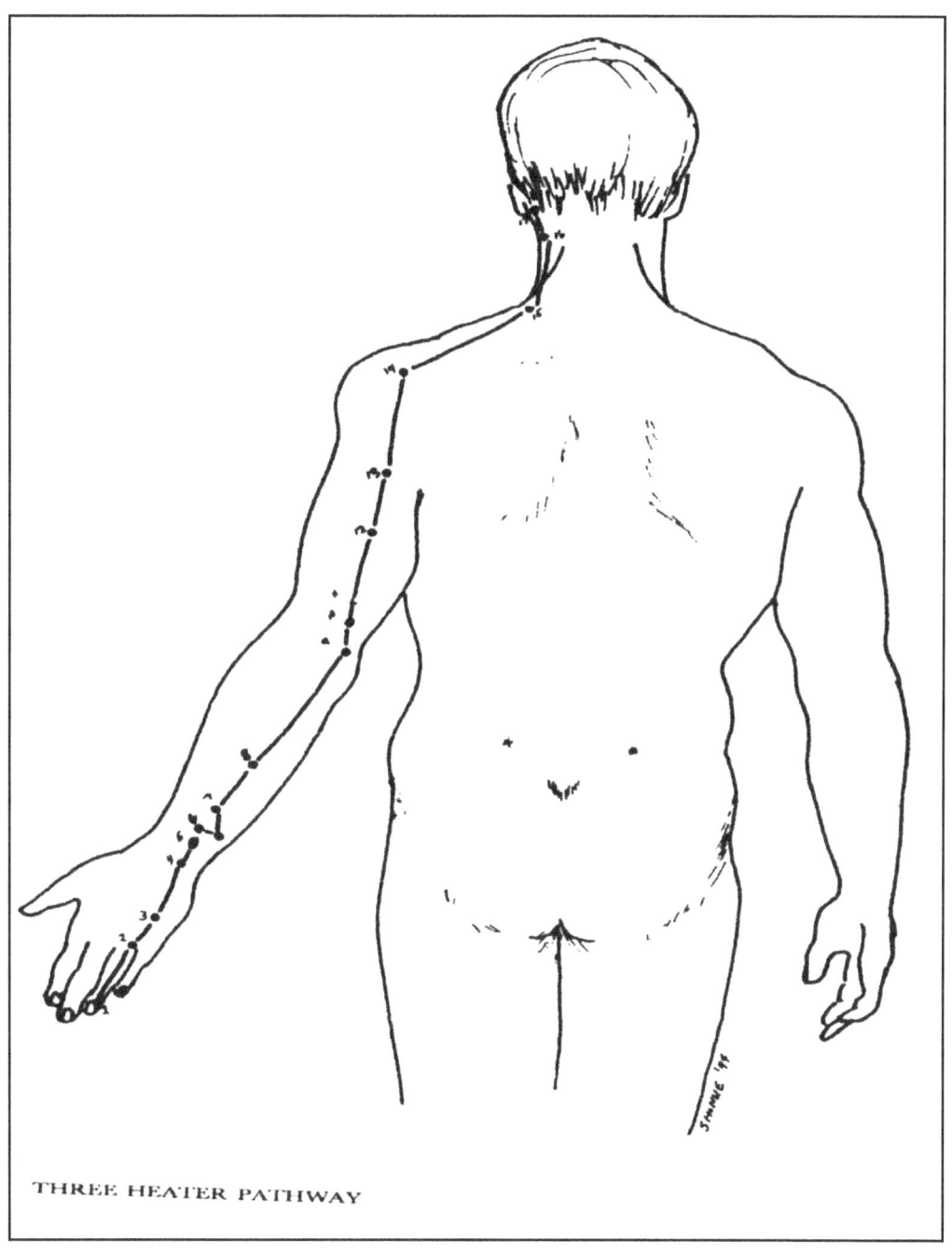

THREE HEATER PATHWAY

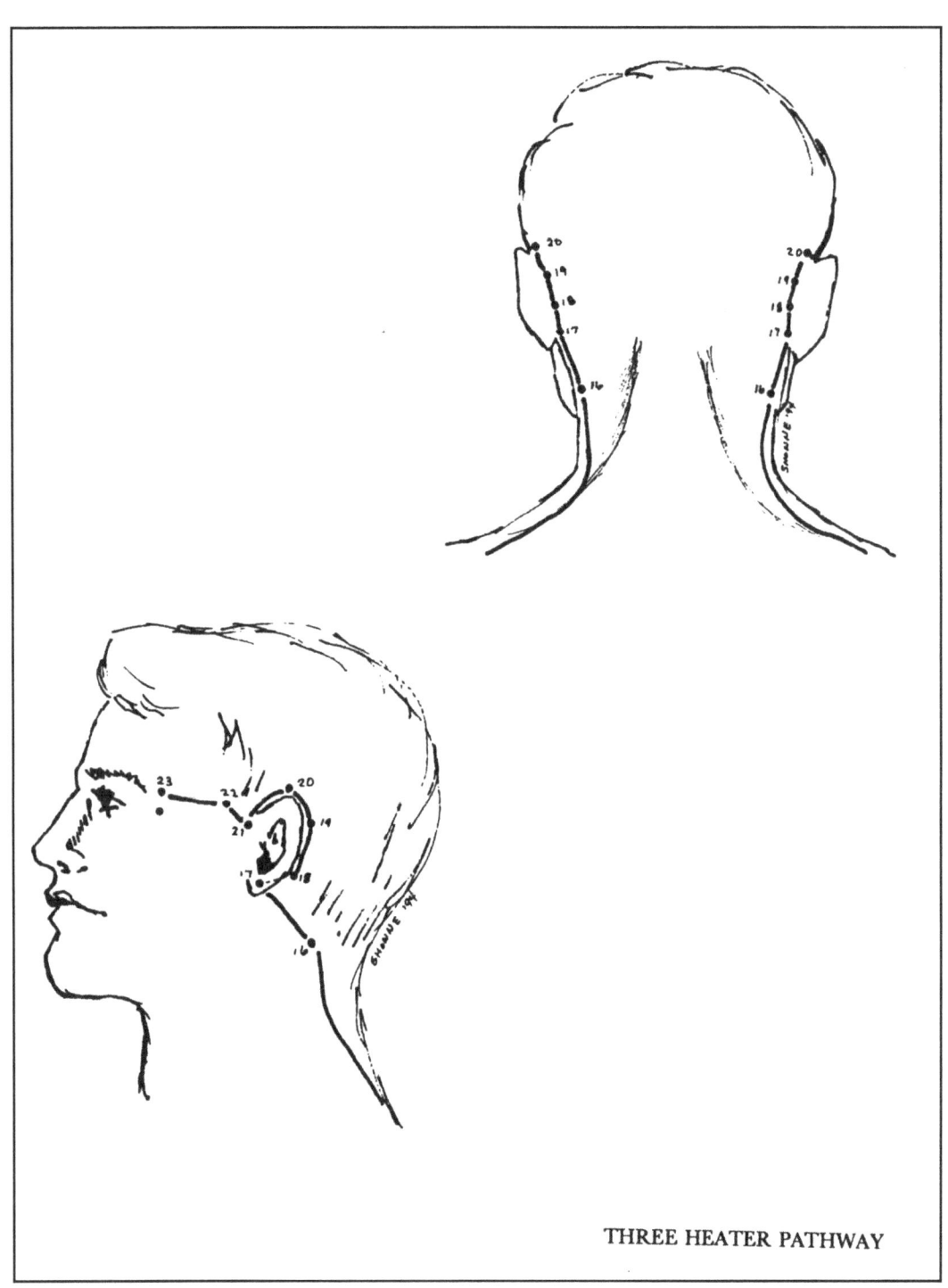

THREE HEATER PATHWAY

THREE HEATER PATHWAY (TH)

TH-l   Rushing the Frontier Gate (metal and entry pts., good pt. for coldness, frigidity, trouble with elbow, unable to raise forearm, frozen shoulder, tennis elbow, numbness)

TH-2 Humor Gate (water pt., good pt. for cold or hot hands and feet, tinnitus, eyes red and painful, mind wanders)

TH-3 Central Islet (wood and tonification pts.; first aid pt: exhaustion, dizziness and lack of balance)

TH-4   Yang Pool (source pt., good pt. for inability to grasp and hold objects, to raise shoulder and bend fingers, also good for improved hearing)

TH-5   Outer Frontier Gate (junction pt., good pt. for difficulty hearing and headaches, ulcers, patient feels that people are a "pain in the neck"; it is a good point for reaching out to others)

TH-6   Branch Ditch (fire, home element, and horary pts., 9 p.m.—11 p.m., good for arthritis and rheumatic conditions)

TH-7   Assembly of Ancestors (a good pt. if you are wondering "Where do I go from here?")

TH-8   Three Yang Connection (meeting pt. for SI, TH and CO; this is good for lack of coordination, pain in the loins, eye diseases, keep this point in mind for a situation when the "body doesn't wish to move")

TH-9   Four Rivers (good pt. for eye disorders, problems with forearm and elbow)

TH-10 Celestial Well (earth and sedation pts.)

TH-11 Pure Cold Abyss

 TH-l2 Relax and Joy

TH-13 Shoulder Meeting

TH-l4 Shoulder Bone Hole

TH-15 Celestial Bone-Hole (first aid pt: colds)

TH-16 Heavenly Window (Window of the Sky)

TH-l7 Wind Screen

TH-18 Spasm Vessel

TH-19 Skull Breathing

TH-20 Small Angle of Ear

TH-21 Ear Gate

TH-22 Harmony Bone-Hole (exit pt.)

TH-23 Silk Bamboo Hollow

CHAPTER 15

TREATMENT PLAN - STOMACH PATHWAY (ST)

Here is a possible treatment plan to work on the stomach (ST) pathway. This plan is immediately followed by point names and locations.

I. If you want to strengthen the ST pathway, you can sting the tonification point (ST-41) or the source point (ST-42).

2. If you want to connect the ST to its paired meridian the spleen (SP), sting yourself on the junction point (ST-40). (See glossary for more information.)

3. You can enhance the effectiveness of your treatment by stinging the home element point (ST-36). This is best done as a horary treatment, which means a treatment on the home element point at the right time of day (7 a.m.— 9 a.m.) and/or in the right season (late summer).

4. If you are having symptoms between 7 a.m.—9 a.m. (i.e., having trouble getting up and getting going, nauseated, or feeling sluggish), then you may want to do acupressure on the entry point (ST-1). This point is forbidden to bee sting, though you can sting the exit point (ST-42). Another reason to consider going to the entry/exit points is if you start to feel better and then you feel like you are going backwards. Your symptoms may go away or are alleviated, and then all of a sudden they return again. Instead of getting discouraged, try treating the entry/exit points!

5. Choose a specific point on the ST based on the name of the point. This is called treating by the spirit of the point. Look at the names of all the points on the ST pathway. Do any of the names jump out at you? What about Hard Bargain (ST-45)? Do you feel like your life is very difficult and it's not fair? Or how about Leg Three Miles (ST-36)? This is a very famous first aid point. It is especially good for nausea, morning sickness, travel sickness. But this point also has another meaning on a spirit level. It is a good point for people who go the extra mile for others, but not for themselves. It's a good point for bringing

nurturing and compassion to some one who needs it. These are just two examples of some of the points on the ST that might speak to you.

6. You may want to consider a Window of the Sky, People Welcome (ST-9). Remember that Windows bring the body, mind, and spirit together. This is a good point for helping someone let people in to their lives and to open up. Since this point is forbidden for bee stings, you will need to use acupressure only.

7. Try combining any of the above recommendations. "BEE" creative. And remember to keep good records.

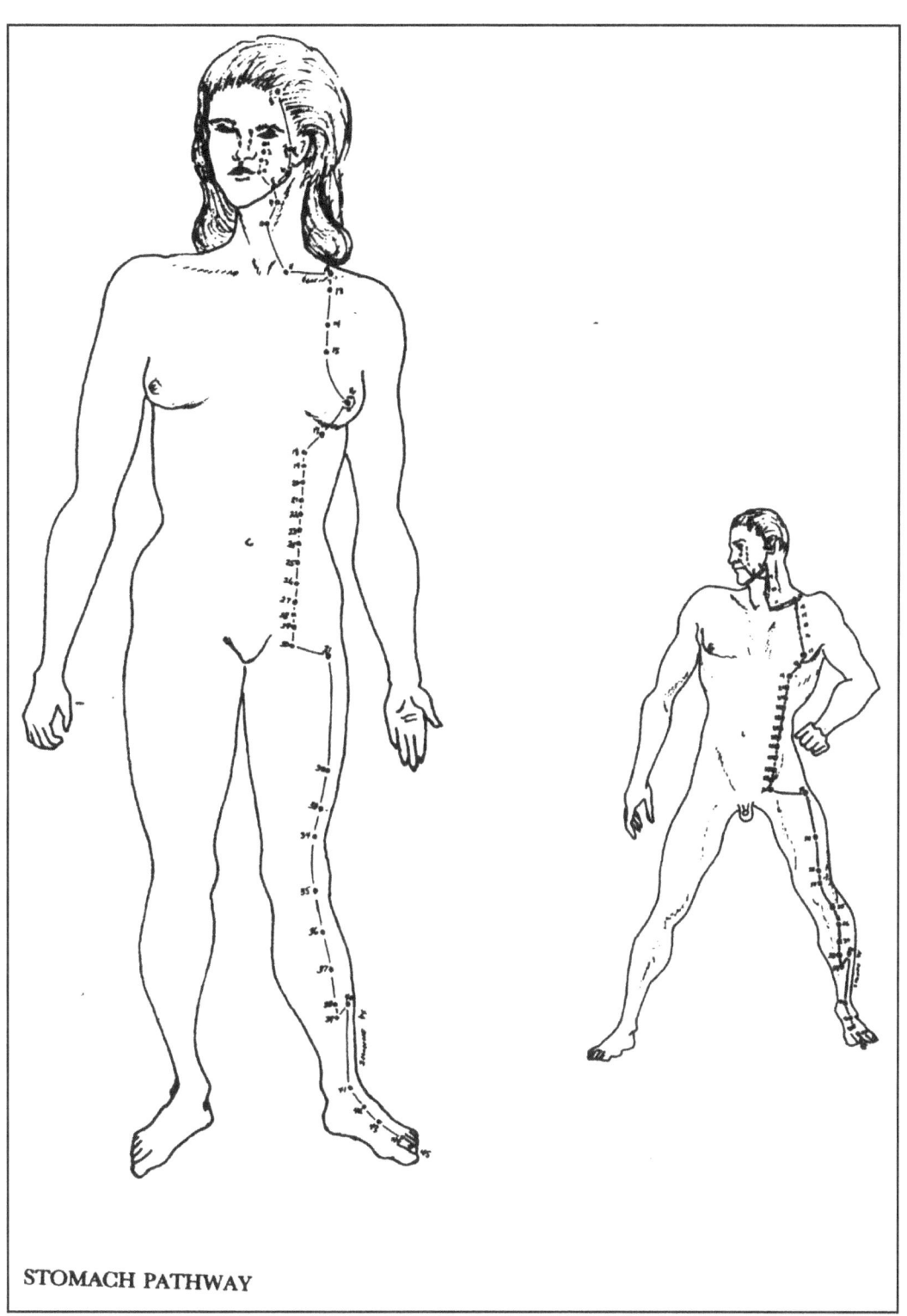

STOMACH PATHWAY

STOMACH PATHWAY

ST-1   Receive Tears, Tear Container (entry pt.)

ST-2   Four Whites (use acupressure only)

ST-3   Great Bone-Hole

ST-4   Earth Granary

ST-5   Great Welcome

ST-6   Jaw Bone

ST-7   Below the Joint

ST-8   Head Corner

ST-9   People Welcome (Window to the Sky. This is a very good spirit pt. for those who need to let people into their lives!)

ST-10 Water Rushing Out

ST-11 Ch'i Cottage (this is a good pt. for energy)

ST-12 Broken Bowl (this spirit pt. is very good for people who feel like their spirit was broken in childhood. They feel like they are Humpty Dumpty, who can't be put back together again)

ST-l3 Ch'i Door (a door to energy)

ST-l4 Storehouse

ST-15 Roof

ST-16 Breast Window

ST-17 Center of the Breasts

ST-18 Root of the Breasts

ST-19 Not at Ease (Good pt. for anxiety)

ST-20 Receiving Fullness

ST-21 Bridge Gate

ST-22 Border Gate

ST-23   Great Oneness (this is a great pt. for those who feel disconnected from others and the universe)

ST-24 Lubrication Food Gate (this is a good pt. for difficulty with food digestion)

ST-25 Celestial Pivot (Internal Dragon pt. and the place within all of us where we meet God)

ST-26 Outside Mound

ST-27 Great Gigantic

ST-28 Water Path

ST-29 The Return

ST-30 Ch'i Rushing (this is a Sea of Nourishment)

ST-3l Thigh Border

ST-32 Prostrate Hare (Internal Dragon pt. and a good pt. for exhaustion, like a rabbit lying by the side of the road)

ST-33 Yin Market

ST-34 Beam Mound

ST-35 Calf's Nose

ST-36 Leg Three Miles (earth, home element, and horary pts., 7 a.m.—9 a.m.; first aid pt: indigestion, fainting and morning sickness. This point is very famous because it is also a Sea of Nourishment and a center of energy.)

ST-37 Upper Great Void

ST-38 Branch Opening (this is a good spirit pt. to create an opening for new ideas or actions! Also good for weakness of legs, inability to move limbs and cold limbs.)

ST-39 Lower Great Void (good for hair coming out in handfuls, rheumatism and arthritis)

ST-40 Abundant Splendor (junction pt. and good spirit pt. for abundance)

ST-41 Released Stream (fire and tonification pts. and Internal Dragon pt.; good for rheumatism and gout)

ST-42 Surging Yang (source and exit pts.)

ST-43 Sunken Valley (wood pt. and a spirit point for a feeling of sinking in quicksand)

ST-44 Inner Courtyard (water pt.)

ST-45 Hard Bargain (metal and sedation pts.; first aid: hangover)

CHAPTER 16

TREATMENT PLAN – SPLEEN PATHWAY (SP)

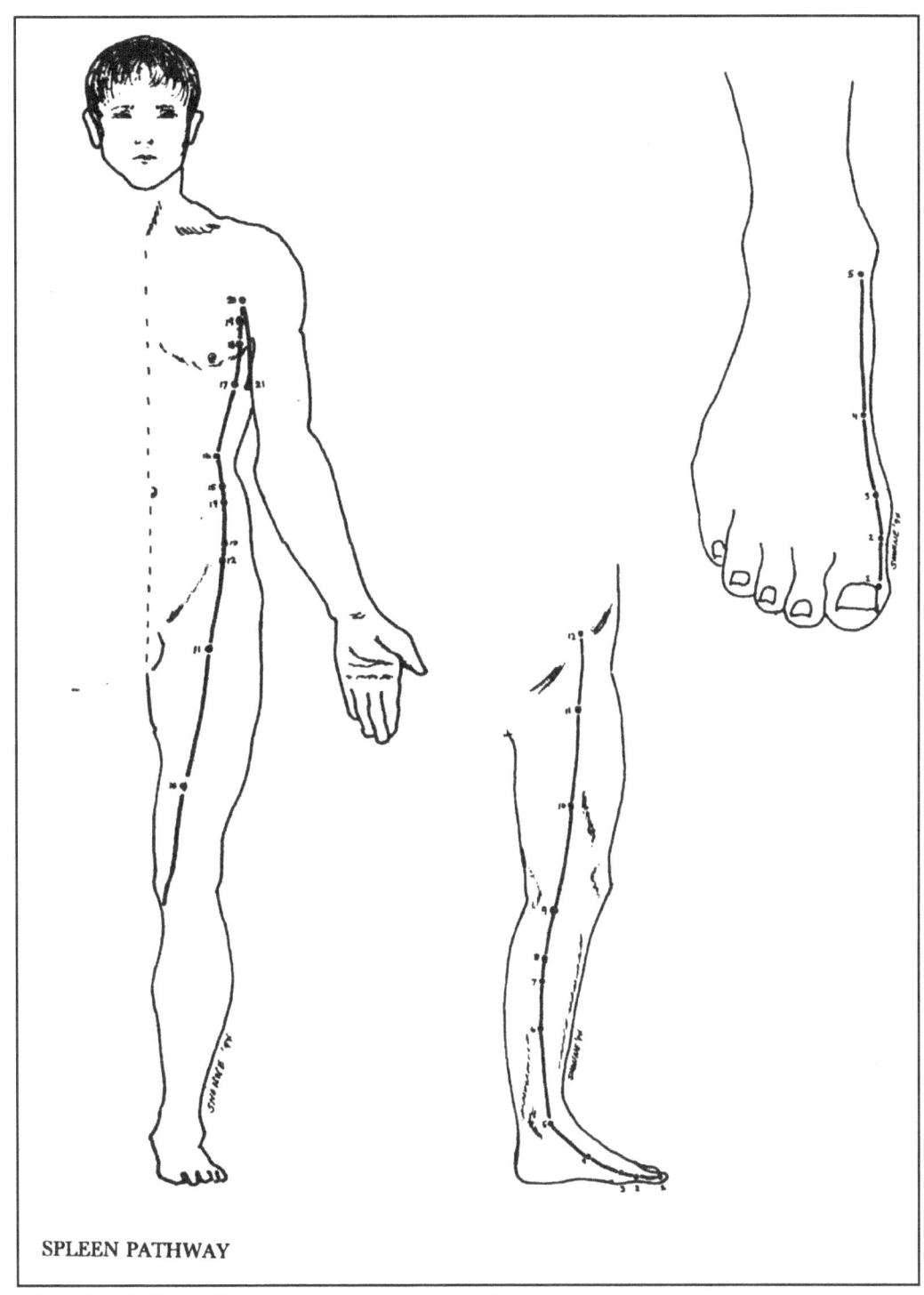

SPLEEN PATHWAY

TREATMENT PLAN - SPLEEN PATHWAY (SP)

Here is a possible treatment plan to work on the spleen (SP) pathway. This plan is immediately followed by point names and locations.

I. If you want to strengthen the SP pathway, you can sting the tonification point (SP-2) or the source point (SP-3).

2. If you want to connect the SP to its paired meridian the stomach (ST), sting yourself on the junction point (SP-4). (See glossary for more information.)

3. You can enhance the effectiveness of your treatment by stinging the home element point (SP-3). This is best done as a horary treatment, which means a treatment on the home element point at the right time of day (9 a.m.— 11 a.m.) and/or in the right season (late summer).

4. If you are having symptoms between 9 a.m.—11 a.m. (i.e., having trouble staying wake, feeling sluggish or depressed), then you may want to sting the entry point (SP-1) and/or the exit point (SP-21). Another reason to consider stinging the entry/exit points is if you start to feel better and then you feel like you are going backwards. Your symptoms may go away or are alleviated, and then all of a sudden they return again. Instead of getting discouraged, try stinging the entry/exit points!

5. Choose a specific point on the SP based on the name of the point. This is called treating by the spirit of the point. Look at the names of all the points on the SP pathway. Do any of the names jump out at you? What about Leaky Valley (SP-7)? Do you ever feel like your energy is leaking out of you? Or how about Earth Motivator (SP-8)? Are you feeling depressed and are you having trouble motivating yourself to do anything? These are just two examples of some of the points on the SP that might speak to you. Also keep good records of your progress.

SPLEEN PATHWAY (SP)

SP-1   Hidden White (wood and entry pts.)

SP-2   Great Metropolis (fire and tonification pts.; first aid pt: fractures and spasms, limbs feel heavy, cold hands and feet)

SP-3   Supreme White, also called "The Mother Within Us that Never Dies" (earth, home element, source and horary pts., 9 a.m.—11 a.m.)

SP-4 Yellow Emperor Prince's Grandson (junction pt. This pt. cured the grandson of the Prince, therefore it may cure you!)

SP-5   Merchant Mound (metal and sedation pts.)

SP-6   Three Yin Intersection (center of energy and a meeting pt. of the Spleen, Kidney, and Liver pathways, good for insomnia and depression)

SP-7   Leaky Valley

SP-8   Earth Motivator (this pt. gets the earth moving)

SP-9   Yin Mound Spring (water pt.)

SP-l0 Sea of Blood

SP-11 Basket Gate

SP-12 Surging Gate

SP-13 Official Residence

SP-14 Abdomen Knot (a good pt. for knots in the abdomen)

SP-15 Great Horizontal

SP-16 Abdomen Sorrow (this is a spirit pt. for sorrow that is so deep it feels like it goes down to the core of your being)

SP-17 Food Drain

SP-18 Celestial Ravine

SP-19 Chest Village

SP-20 Encircling Glory

SP-21 Great Enveloping (exit pt. and spirit pt. for feeling nurtured and enveloped by motherly love and compassion)

CHAPTER 17

TREATMENT PLAN - LUNG PATHWAY (L)

Here is a possible treatment plan to work on the lung (L) pathway. This plan is immediately followed by point names and locations.

   I. If you want to strengthen the L pathway, you can sting the tonification point (L-9) or the source point (L-9).

   2. If you want to connect the L to its paired meridian the colon (CO), sting yourself on the junction point (L-7). (See glossary for more information.)

   3. You can enhance the effectiveness of your treatment by stinging the home element point (L-8). This is best done as a horary treatment, which means a treatment on the home element point at the right time of day (3 a.m.—5 a.m.) and/or in the right season (autumn).

   4. If you are having symptoms between 3 a.m.—5 a.m. (i.e., waking up at that time every night), then you may want to sting the entry point (L-1) and/or the exit point (L-7). Another reason to consider stinging the entry/exit points is if you start to feel better and then you feel like you are going backwards. Your symptoms may go away or are alleviated, and then all of a sudden they return again. Instead of getting discouraged, try stinging the entry/exit points!

   5. Choose a specific point on the L based on the name of the point. This is called treating by the spirit of the point. Look at the names of all the points on the L pathway. Do any of the names jump out at you? What about Greatest Hole (L-6)? Do you ever feel like you are in a very deep hole and you cannot get out? Or how about Narrow Defile (L-7)? Do you ever feel like you barely have room to move? It's like being "between a rock and a hard place?" These are just two examples of some of the points on the L that might speak to you.

   6. There is also a Window of the Sky on the L pathway (L-3). This would also be a good spirit point to work out your relationship you're your father and your Heavenly Father.

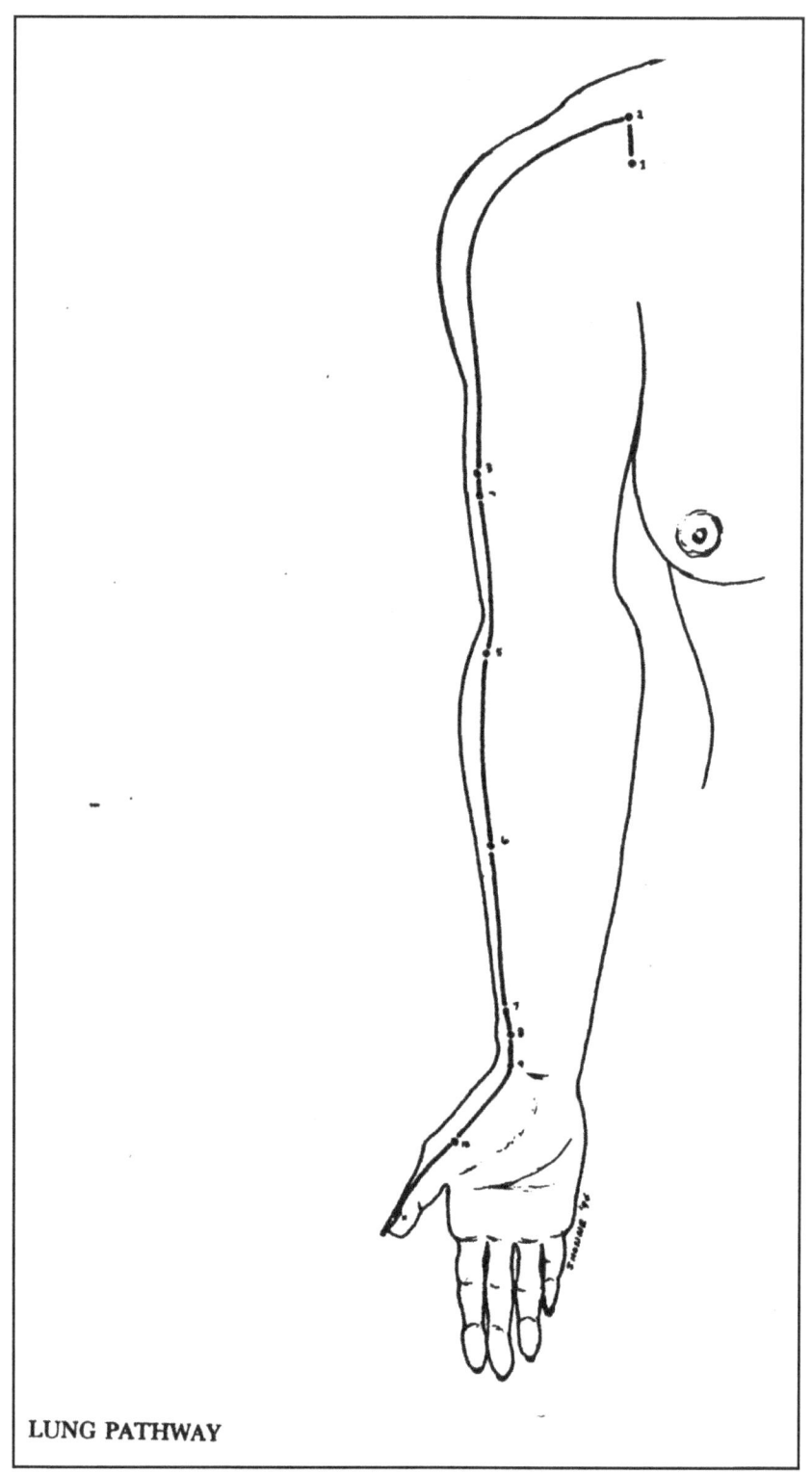

LUNG PATHWAY

LUNG PATHWAY (L)

L-l   Central Treasury (entry pt., first aid pt: drowning)

L-2   Cloud Gate (this is a very spiritual pt.)

L-3   Celestial Storehouse (Window of the Sky)

L-4   Guarding White

L-5   Outside Marsh (water and sedation pts.)

L-6 Greatest Hole (very good pt. for deep depression, fear, tension headaches and elbow trouble)

L-7   Narrow Defile (junction and exit pts. A good spirit pt. if you are stuck "between a rock and a hard place," or are repeating an experience over and over again; good for skin disorders, ice cold limbs and bones.)

L-8   Meridian Gutter (metal, home element, and horary pts., 3 a.m.—5 a.m., first aid pt: electric shock. This is a wonderful pt. in the autumn, especially if the person is dreaming about death or has a fear of dying. This pt. is good when heat and cold are all out of proportion in the hands.)

L-9   Very Great Abyss, the Grand Canyon Pt. (earth, tonification and source pts., first aid pt. for shock and asphyxia, cold hands and feet, can't grasp objects, loss of sensations in fingers, insomnia; facial neuralgia. This is a good spirit pt. for feeling like you are in a deep, dark hole. You can see everyone else up there in the light but you feel like you can't get there.)

L-10   Fish Border (fire pt. This pt. will warm up the metal in the body so it is good for rigidity, good for asthma and hayfever)

L-11 Little Merchant (wood pt. and first aid pt: convulsions, sunstroke, numbness of the hands and arms)

CHAPTER 18

TREATMENT PLAN - COLON PATHWAY

Here is a possible treatment plan to work on the colon (CO) pathway. This plan is immediately followed by point names and locations.

I. If you want to strengthen the CO pathway, you can sting the tonification point (CO-11) or the source point (CO-4).

2. If you want to connect the CO to its paired meridian the lung (L), sting yourself on the junction point (CO-6).

3. You can enhance the effectiveness of your treatment by stinging the home element point (CO-1). This is best done as a horary treatment, which means a treatment on the home element point at the right time of day (5 a.m.—7 a.m.) and/or in the right season (autumn).

4. If you are having symptoms between 5 a.m.—7 a.m. (i.e., waking up at that time every morning), then you may want to sting the entry point (CO-4) and/or use acupressure on the exit point (CO-20). Another reason to consider entry/exit points is if you start to feel better and then you feel like you are going backwards. Your symptoms may go away or are alleviated, and then all of a sudden they return again. Instead of getting discouraged, try treating the entry/ exit points!

5. Choose a specific point on the CO based on the name of the point. This is called treating by the spirit of the point. Look at the names of all the points on the CO pathway. Do any of the names jump out at you? What about "The Great Letting Go," also called Union Valley (CO-4)? Does that sound like you? Do you have trouble letting go of the past? Or what about Shoulder Bone (CO-15)? That might be a good point if you are having shoulder or arm problems. These are just two examples of some of the points on the CO that might speak to you.

6. You could also do a Window to the Sky, Support and Rush Out (CO-18). This will bring the body, mind, and spirit together. This is a great spirit point for surrendering to the universe and going with the flow.

7. Try combining any of the above recommendations. "BEE" creative.

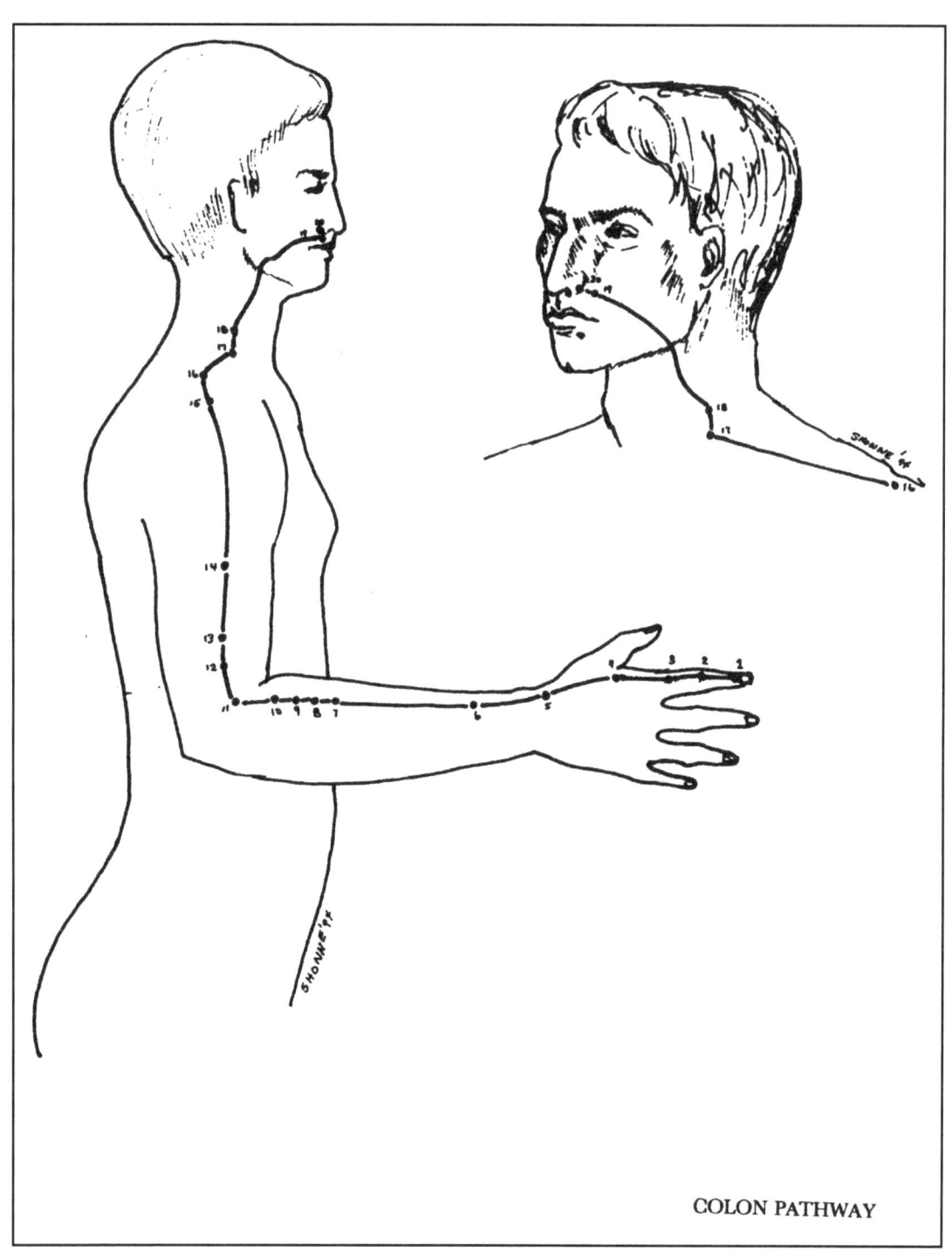

COLON PATHWAY

97

COLON (CO) ALSO CALLED THE LARGE INTESTINE (LI)

CO-l Merchant Yang (metal, home element, and horary pts., 5 a.m.—7 a.m., as well as first aid pt: toothache, frozen shoulder, neck problems)

CO-2 Second Space (water and sedation pts., good pt. for rigidity or feeling bone dry, inability to lift arm)

CO-3 Third Space (wood pt.)

CO-4 Union Valley, also known as "The Great Letting Go" (entry and source pts. as well as a center of energy; first aid pt: dull pains, earache, fainting, headaches, and spots in front of eyes, food poisoning, poison, and toothache. This is an important spirit pt. for letting go of the past!)

CO-5 Yang Stream (fire pt., good pt. for tinnitus, deafness)

CO-6 Side Passage (junction pt.)

CO-7 Warm Flow (good pt. for a patient who feels there's "no good in life," speech difficulties)

CO-8 Lower Ridge (good for headaches, speech problems)

CO-9 Upper Ridge (good for brain fatigue, arthritic knee, paralysis, loss of sensation of limbs)

CO-10 Arm Three Miles (good for rheumatism, arthritis, trouble bending and raising arms, goiters)

CO-11 Pool at the Bend (earth and tonification pts. This is a very good pt. for tennis elbow and arm problems, toothaches, eye problems, pleurisy, asthma, hayfever, bronchitis.)

CO-12 Elbow Bone

CO-13 Arm Five Miles

CO-14 Outer Bone of the Arm

CO-15 Shoulder Bone (first aid pt.: shoulder, concussion, electric shock, exhaustion, shock, and head injury)

CO-I6 Great Bone

CO-I7 Celestial Tripod

CO-I8 Support and Rush Out (Window of the Sky and a good spirit pt. for surrendering to a Higher Power and letting things go)

CO-I9 Grain Bone-Hole (use acupressure only)

CO-20 Welcome Fragrance (exit pt. and good pt for sinus problems, allergies, and clogged nose)

CHAPTER 19

TREATMENT PLAN - BLADDER PATHWAY

Here is a possible treatment plan to work on the bladder (BL) pathway. This plan is immediately followed by point names and locations.

l. If you want to strengthen the BL pathway, you can sting the tonification point (BL-67) or the source point (BL-64). (See glossary for more information.)

2. If you want to connect the BL to its paired meridian the kidney (K), sting yourself on the junction point (BL-58).

3. You can enhance the effectiveness of your treatment by stinging the home element point (BL-66). This is best done as a horary treatment, which means a treatment on the home element point at the right time of day (3 p.m.—5 p.m.) and/or in the right season (winter).

4. If you are having symptoms every day between 3 p.m.—5 p.m. (i.e., a consistent pattern of feeling very tired, like someone just "pulled the plug"), then you may want to use acupressure on the entry point (BL-1), since it is forbidden to sting this point. You can sting the exit point (BL-67). Another reason to consider using the entry/exit points is if you start to feel better and then you feel like you are going backwards. Your symptoms may go away or are alleviated, and then all of a sudden they return again. Instead of getting discouraged, try treating the entry/exit points!

5. Choose a specific point on the BL based on the name of the point. This is called treating by the spirit of the point. Look at the names of all the points on the BL pathway. Do any of the names jump out at you? What about Fly and Scatter (BL-58)? Does that sound like you? Are you feeling scattered and do you need a little peace and quiet? This is just one example of some of the points on the BL that might speak to you.

6. Or how about a Window of the Sky, Celestial Pillar (BL-10)? This point will help to bring the body, mind, and spirit together. Even the

name of the point makes you think of a heavenly pillar standing straight and tall.

7. Try combining any of the above recommendations. "BEE" creative.

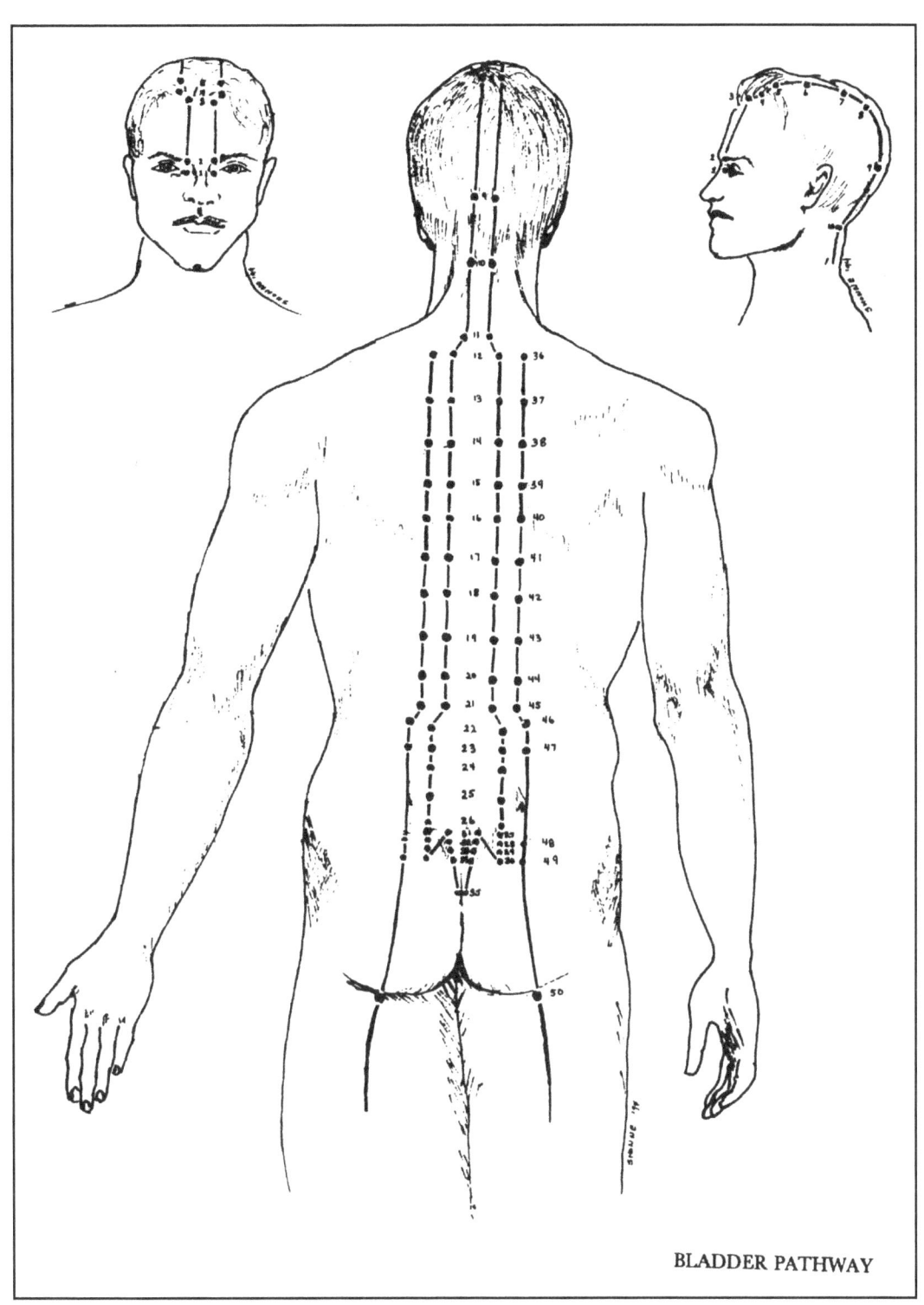

BLADDER PATHWAY

102

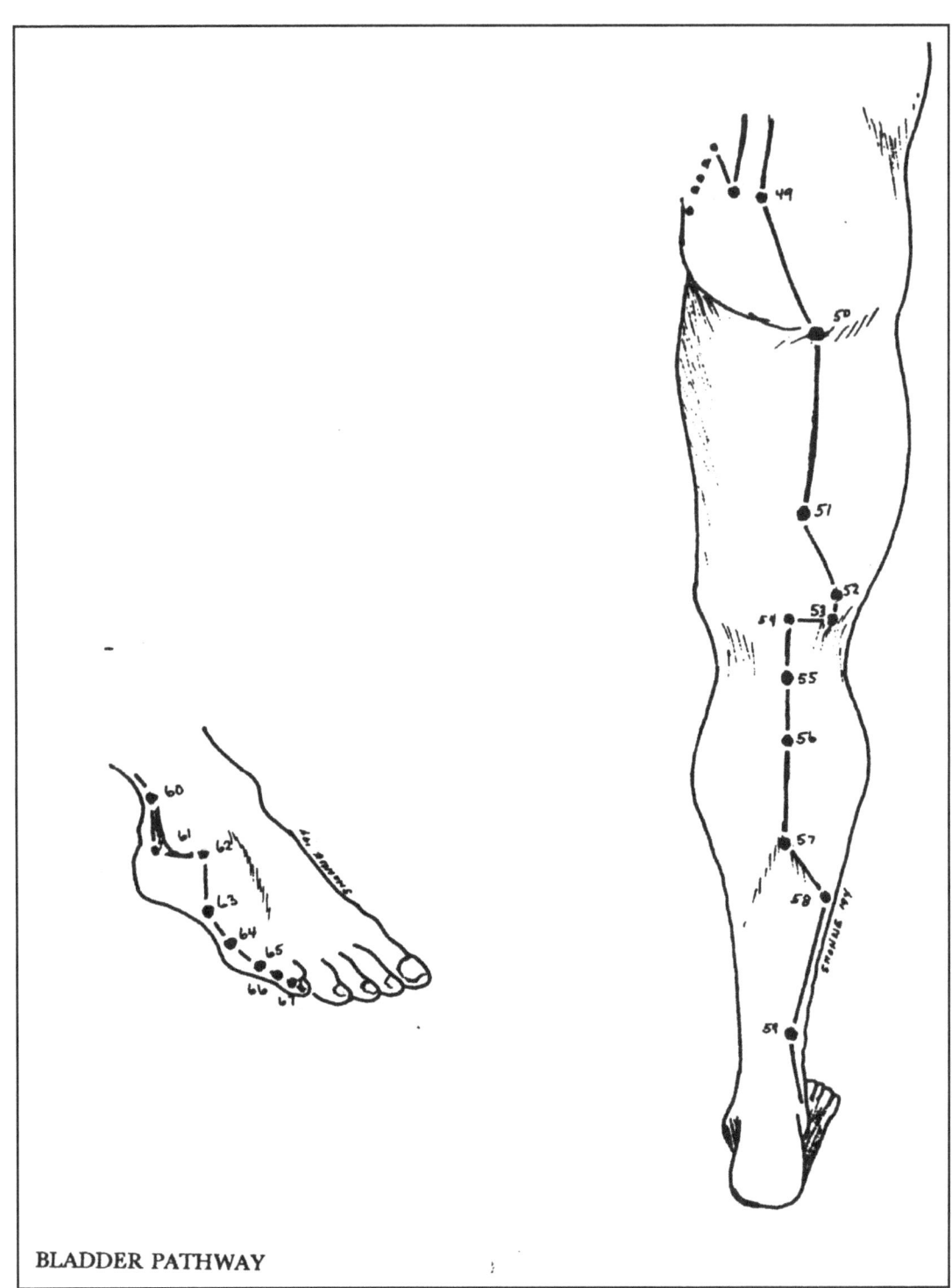

BLADDER PATHWAY

BLADDER PATHWAY (BL)

BL-1   Bright Eyes (entry pt.)

BL-2   Bamboo Gathering

BL-3   Eyebrows Rushing

BL-4   Deviating Turn

BL-5   Five Places

BL-6   Receive Light

BL-7   Celestial Connection

BL-8   Declining Connection Luo End

BL-9   Jade Pillow

BL-10   Celestial Pillar (Window of the Sky)

BL-11   Great Shuttle (External Dragon pt., first aid pt: fractures and sprains)

BL-l2   Wind Gate

BL-l3   Lung Shu

BL-l4   Heart Protector Shu

BL-l5   Heart Shu

BL-l6   Governor Shu

BL-l7   Diaphragm Shu

BL-18   Liver Shu

BL-l9 Gall Bladder Shu

BL-20 Spleen Shu

BL-21 Stomach Shu

BL-22 Three Heater Shu

BL-23 Kidney Shu

BL-24 Sea of Ch'i Shu

BL-25 Colon Shu

BL-26 First Gate Shu

BL-27 Small Intestine Shu

BL-28 Bladder Shu

BL-29 Central Backbone Shu

BL-30 White Ring Shu

BL-3l Upper Bone-Hole

BL-32 Second Bone-Hole

BL-33 Central Bone-Hole

BL-34 Lower Bone-Hole

BL-35 Meeting of Yang

BL-36 Near Division

BL-37 Soul Door or Gate of Abundance (spirit pt. for the Lungs)

BL-38 Superficial Cleft, also known as The Happy Point (spirit pt. for Heart Protector)

BL-39 Bend Yang (spirit pt. for the Heart)

BL-40 Wail of Grief

BL-41 Diaphragm Border

BL-42 Spiritual Soul Gate (spirit pt. for the Liver)

BL-43 Yang Net (spirit pt. for the Gall Bladder)

BL-44 Thought Dwelling (spirit pt. for the Spleen)

BL-45 Stomach Granary (spirit pt. for the Stomach)

BL-46 Diaphragm Gate of Vitality (spirit pt. for the Three Heater)

BL-47 Ambition Room (spirit pt. for the Kidneys)

BL-48 Womb and Heart Diaphragm (spirit pt. for the Bladder)

BL-49 Orderly Frontier

BL-50 Receive and Support (good first aid pt. for muscles)

BL-51 Prosperous Gate

BL-52 Floating Reserve

BL-53 Equilibrium Yang

BL-54 Equilibrium Middle (earth pt., first aid pt: spinal injury, skin diseases, arthritis of knee, night sweats, and stiff neck)

BL-55 Uniting Yang

BL-56 Supporting Muscles

BL-57 Supporting Mountain

BL-58 Fly and Scatter, Taking Flight (junction pt., good pt. to calm down; center of energy pt., good first aid pt. for strengthening vitality, also good for weakness of legs, cystitis, constipation, and lumbago)

BL-59 Instep Yang (first aid pt: food poisoning, elimination of toxins, both physical and mental)

BL-60 Kunlun Mountain (fire pt., first aid pt.: anxiety, facial neuralgia, fractures, spinal injury, sprains; inability to do things, can't turn neck and elbow, swelling of feet and hands, glandular disease, sciatica. This pt. is good for fear in relationships.)

BL-61 Servant's Aide (External Dragon's pt., first aid pt. for pain in knee, spasm in calf, can't raise the knee, needs help up stairs and getting in car)

BL-62 Extended Meridian (good pt. for diseases of the spine)

BL-63 Metal Gate (good pt. for swelling, tinnitus)

BL-64 Capital Bone (source pt., first aid pt: bee stings, stiff neck, lumbago, red eyes)

BL-65 Bone Binder (wood, sedation pts., first aid pt: burns, cystitis, food poisoning, insect bites, poison, scalds, sunburn, urine retention and frequency, difficulty healing a bone, fear of wind and cold, sciatica)

BL-66 Penetrating Valley (water, home element, and horary pts., 3 p.m.-5 p.m., good pt. for blurred vision, dreams of drowning and falling, fear of the unknown, worrying about "What's going to happen next?," stiffness in neck, pain in feet and calves, edema)

BL-67 Reaching Yin (metal, tonification, and exit pts.)

CHAPTER 20

TREATMENT PLAN - KIDNEY PATHWAY

Here is a possible treatment plan to work on the kidney (K) pathway. This plan is immediately followed by point names and locations.

I. If you want to strengthen the K pathway, you can sting the tonification point (K-7) or the source point (K-3).

2. If you want to connect the K to its paired meridian the bladder (BL), sting yourself on the junction point (K-4). (See glossary for more information.)

3. You can enhance the effectiveness of your treatment by stinging the home element point (K-10). This is best done as a horary treatment, which means a treatment on the home element point at the right time of day (5 p.m.- 7 p.m.) and/or in the right season (winter).

4. If you are having symptoms every day between 5 p.m.-7 p.m. (i.e., feeling very tired or feeling like someone has "just pulled the plug"), then you may want to sting the entry point (K-1) and/or the exit point (K-22). If you have trouble finding this point on a woman you can also use K-27. Another reason to consider stinging the entry/exit points is if you start to feel better and then you feel like you are going backwards. Your symptoms may go away or are alleviated, and then all of a sudden they return again. Instead of getting discouraged, try stinging the entry/exit points!

5. Choose a specific point on the K based on the name of the point. This is called treating by the spirit of the point. Look at the names of all the points on the K pathway. Do any of the names jump out at you? What about Spirit Burial Ground (K- 24)? This is a wonderful point for resurrecting the spirit in someone after they feel that a part of them has died. Does that sound like you? Or how about Shining Sea (K-6)? This is like looking in a pond of water, seeing your reflection, and gaining insight from what you see. These are just two examples of some of the points on the K that might speak to you.

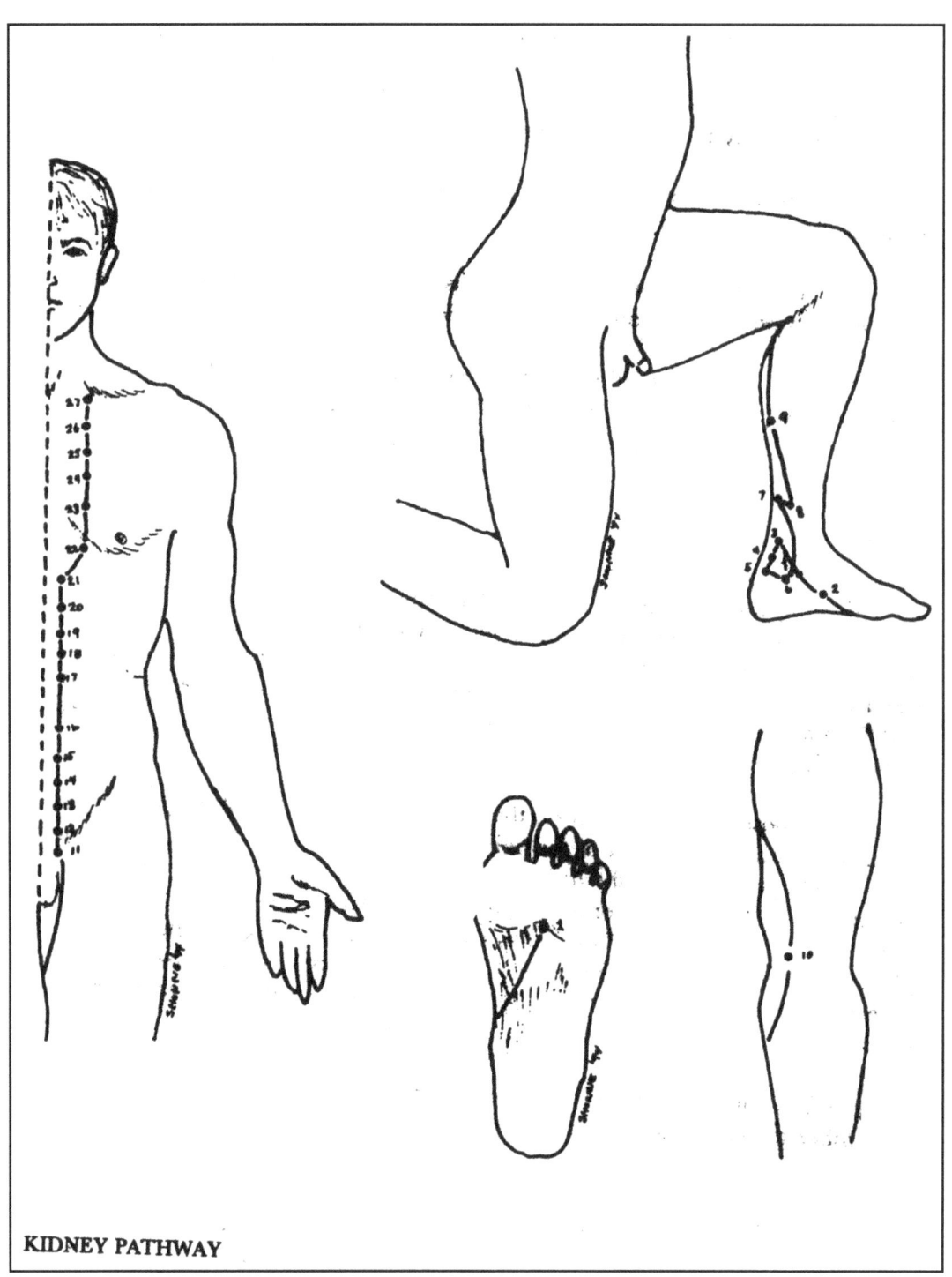

KIDNEY PATHWAY

KIDNEY PATHWAY (K)

K-l Gushing Spring (wood, sedation, and entry pts., first aid pt: retention of fluid and beet red face)

K-2 Blazing Valley (fire pt., first aid pt: cystitis, night sweats and impotence)

K-3 Greater Mountain Stream (earth and source pts., first aid pt: dryness, sore throat, insomnia, migraines, epilepsy, irregular menses, limbs weary and heavy)

K-4 Large Goblet (junction pt., first aid pt: blurred vision, depression before period)

K-5 Water Spring (first aid pt: problems with base of the spine, fear and depression together, agoraphobia)

K-6 Shining Sea (first aid pt: bee stings, concussion, very dark urine and pains in chest; a good spirit pt. for illumination)

K-7 Recover Flow (metal and tonification pts., lots of sweating or none at all)

K-8 Exchange Pledges (menstrual disorders, uterus prolapse)

K-9 Guest House (weakness in legs, spasms, twitches)

K-l0 Yin Valley (water, home element, and horary pts., 5 p.m.—
7 p.m. first aid pt: excessive perspiration, vaginal discharge, depression, watering eyes, pain around genitals, swollen painful abdomen)

K-11 Pubic Bone

K-l2 Great Brightness

K-l3 Door of Infants (center of energy pt.)

K-l4 Four Full

K-l5 Middle Flowing Out

K-l6 Vitals Correspondence

K-17 Merchant Crooked

K-l8 Stone Pass

K-l9 Yin Capital

K-20 Open Valley

K-21 Dark Gate

K-22 Walking on the Veranda (exit pt.; picture yourself walking on a veranda)

K-23 Spirit Seal (first aid pt.- sunstroke. This is a spirit pt. to help you remember who you really are and what you came here to do.)

K-24 Spirit Burial Ground, Spirit Ruins (a great pt. to resurrect the spirit, after a part of you has died)

K-25 Spirit Storehouse

K-26 Amidst Elegance

K-27 Storehouse

CHAPTER 21

TREATMENT PLAN - CONCEPTION VESSEL (CV) – REN MERIDIAN

This pathway is not ruled by the five elements. The conception vessel is part of the 8 extra meridians. Here are some possible reasons why you might want to use the CV:

I. This pathway is the most yin pathway in the body. Go to this pathway if you need to go inward, go home. This pathway will bring someone into themselves.

2. Go to this pathway if you are doing pretty well but just need a little push in the right direction.

Here are some possible points you can use on the conception vessel:

I. If someone has a cold lower abdomen and/or is trying to get pregnant, this is a good point (CV-4), First Gate.

2. CV-3 (Central Pole) is a good point for the bladder and a center of energy.

3. CV-6 (Sea of Ch'i) is a good point to bring nourishment.

4. CV-8 (Spirit Tower Gate) is a wonderful point to build up someone's spirit. May relate to birth trauma. This is the umbilicus, so take care here. I wouldn't do this pt. very early in treatment due to possible swelling.

5. If you have had a severe blow to the top of the head or the very base of the spine, you may want to do the entry/exit points for CV and GV with acupressure or perhaps bee stings (CV-1, CV-24; GV-1, GV-28).

6. Choose a specific point on the pathway based on the name of the point. This is called treating by the spirit of the point. Look at all the names of points on the list for the CV. Do any of those names jump out

at you? For example, what about Stone Gate (CV-5)? Do you sometimes feel like you are banging your head against a wall? Is there a stone in the way that prevents you from getting out of the gate? Then you may want to consider Stone Gate. What about Chest Center (CV-17)? Do you carry everything within? Does this sound like you? These are just two examples of some of the points on the CV that might speak to you.

7. Consider going to a Window of the Sky, Celestial Chimney (CV-22). Remember that Windows bring the body, mind, and spirit together. This is a very helpful point for people who have trouble receiving love and compassion. If you don't want to do a bee sting on this point, you can use gentle pressure.

8. Try combining any of the above recommendations. "BEE" creative. And remember to keep good records.

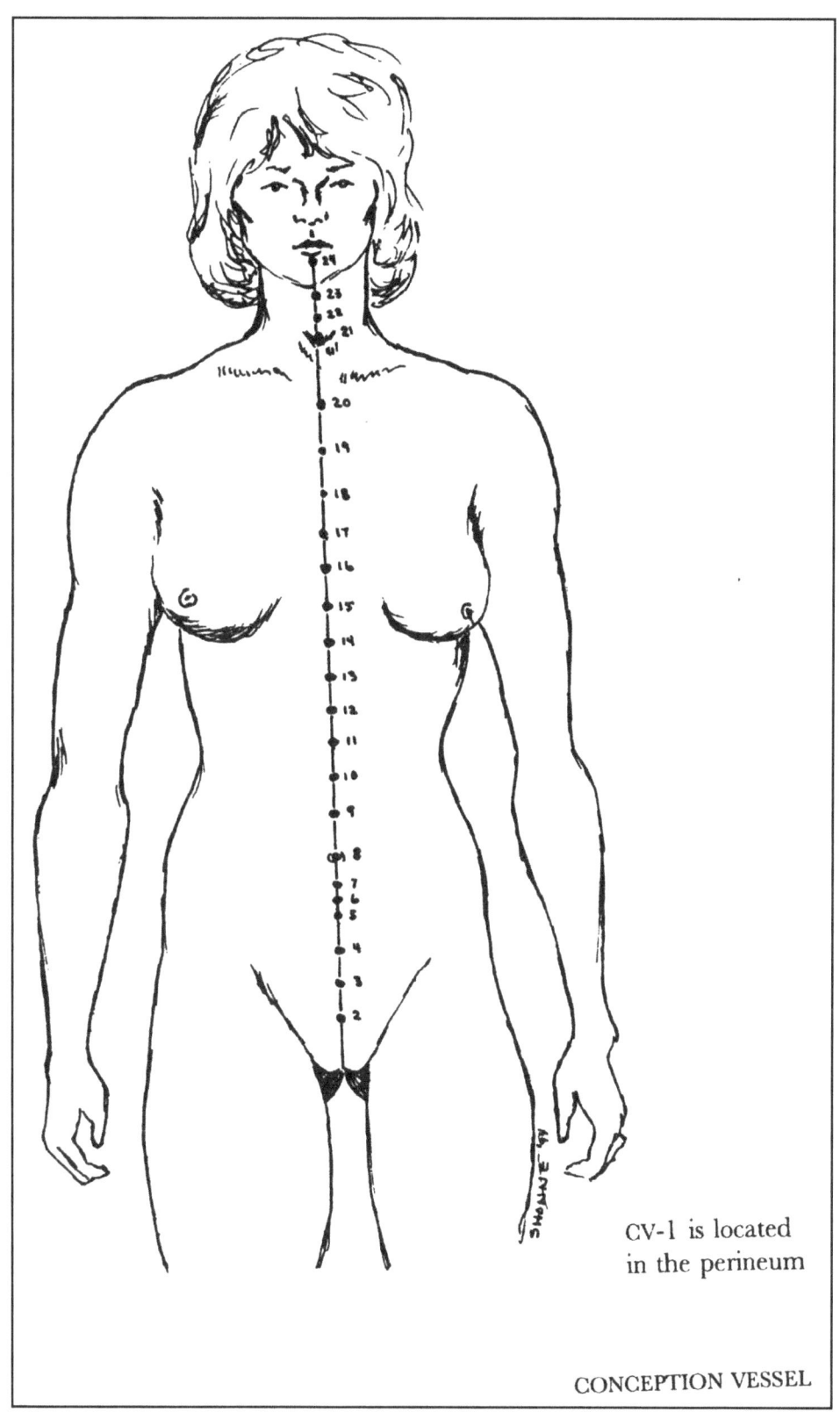

CV-1 is located
in the perineum

CONCEPTION VESSEL

CONCEPTION VESSEL (CV) – REN MERIDIAN

CV-I Meeting of Yin (entry pt. and first aid pt.: drowning. This is a spirit pt. For feeling like you're drowning in a sea of emotions. This point is located in the perineum; you may want to use only acupressure.)

CV-2 Curved Bone (good for impotence)

CV-3 Central Pole (center of energy and first aid pt: urinary problems)

CV-4 Origin Pass (center of energy and this pt. can affect the small intestine, also good for infertility; forbidden during pregnancy)

CV-5 Stone Gate (main center of energy, a pt. related to the three heater pathway and body temperature, good for infertility; forbidden in pregnancy)

CV-6 Sea of Ch'i (main center of energy)

CV-7 Yin Intersection (affects warmth in the lower abdomen, good for infertility and menstrual disorders)

CV-8 Spirit Tower Gate (great spirit pt. for birth trauma and loneliness)

CV-9 Water Divide

CV-10 Lower Venter (forbidden in pregnancy)

CV-11 Interior Strengthening (good for edema)

CV-12 Middle Venter (center of energy)

CV-I3 Upper Venter

CV-I4 Great Tower Gate (affects the heart and first aid for sea and travel sickness)

CV-15 Dove Tail (Internal Dragon pt. and an alarm pt. for the heart protector)

CV-16 Central Palace

CV-l7 Chest Center (sea of energy and a pt. affecting breathing)

CV-18 Jade Hall

CV-l9 Purple Palace

CV-20 Flower Covering

CV-21 Jade Pivot

CV-22 Celestial Chimney (Window of the Sky, a spirit pt. for those who have trouble receiving love and support) You can use gentle pressure here if you don't want to do a bee sting.

CV-23 Ridge Spring (You can use gentle acupressure.)

CV-24 Receiving Fluid (exit pt.)

CHAPTER 22

TREATMENT PLAN - GOVERNOR VESSEL (GV) or DU MERIDIAN

The Governor Vessel (GV) is not ruled by the five elements. It is part of the 8 extra meridians. Here are some possible reasons why you might want to go to the GV:

l. It is the most predominantly yang pathway in the body. It is like sunlight and connects you with the heavens. It is outwardly moving and is filled with powerful energy.

2. This pathway will tend to bring someone outside of themselves.

3. This is a good pathway to go to if you are doing pretty well, but you need a little push in the right direction, in this case out into the world.

Here are some possible points you can use on the Governor Vessel:

l. A good first aid point for concussions, fractures, and spinal injuries is Lumbar Yang Pass (GV-3).

2. Contracted Muscle (GV-8) is good for tight muscles.

3. Meeting of 1000 Ancestors (GV-20) is a very good point for epilepsy and just calming the spirit in general.

4. If you've had a severe blow to the top of the head or the very base of the spine, you can use acupressure or bee stings on the entry/exit points on CV and GV.

5. Choose a specific point on the GV based on the name of the point. This is called treating by the spirit of the point. Look at the names of all the points on the GV. Do any of the names jump out at you? What about Gate of Life (GV-4)? This is for people who are not open to life. This point gives them a little push outward. (GV-4 is forbidden to sting for people under the age of 20.) Are you feeling depressed or hopeless? Do you feel like nothing is ever going to change? Consider this point: It will push you into your destiny. Now, look at Body Pillar

(GV-12). Go to this point when there is no backbone on the body, mind, spirit level. You might feel like you're "crumbling." This point is very good for someone who gets sick a lot and has no center. It is also helpful for someone who is too rigid. And don't forget about GV-14, Great Hammer! This is a great point for hitting someone over the head and pushing them in the direction in which they are already going. These are just three examples of some of the points on the GV that might speak to you.

6. You might also want to consider a Window of the Sky, Wind Mansion (GV- 16). Keep in mind that Windows bring the body, mind and spirit together. This point will bring you closer to the heavens if you are shut down (if your Window is closed) or it can close your Window if it is too open (you are not grounded).

7. Try combining any of the above recommendations. "BEE" creative.

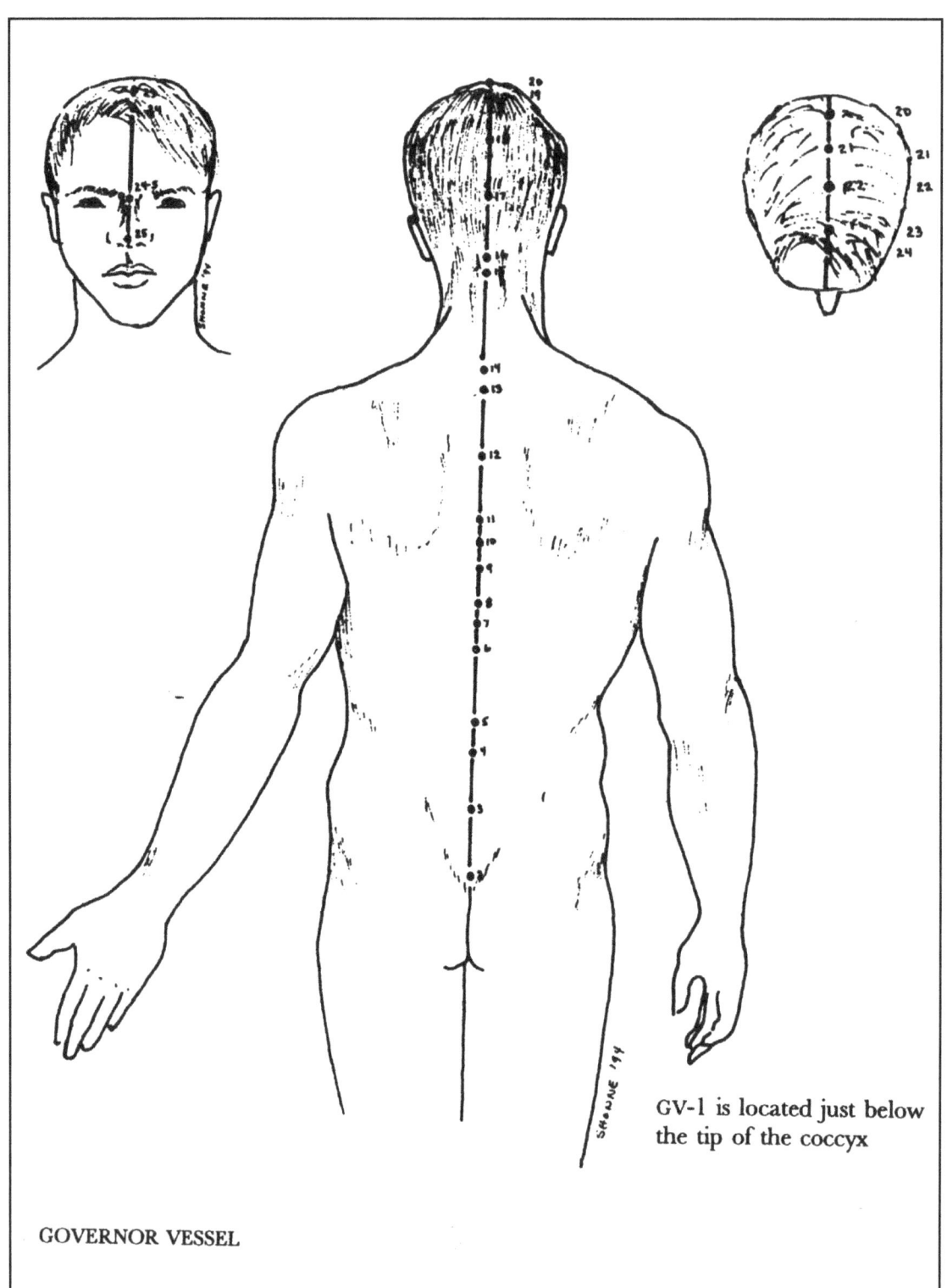

GV-1 is located just below
the tip of the coccyx

GOVERNOR VESSEL

119

GOVERNOR VESSEL (GV) – DU MERIDIAN

GV-1   Long Strong (entry pt. This point is located just below the coccyx.)

GV-2   Lumbar Shu

GV-3   Lumbar Yang Pass (first aid pt.: concussion, fractures, sprains, and spinal injury)

GV-4   Gate of Life (spirit pt. to bring someone back to life)

GV-5   Suspended Pivot (good pt. for rigidity and stiffness)

GV-6   Middle of the Spine

GV-7   Central Pivot

GV-8   Contracted Muscle (This is a good pt. for muscle spasms.)

GV-9   Utmost Yang

GV-10 Spirit Tower

GV-11 Spirit Path

GV-12 Body Pillar (good pt. for strength and standing straight, good for rheumatic diseases)

GV-13 Kiln Path (good for rigid shoulders)

GV-14 Great Hammer (reunion pt. for the following pathways: SI, BL, TH, GB, CO, ST and GV. Also a first aid pt. for colds. This is a spirit pt. when someone needs to be hit over the head with a hammer to get them moving in the right direction. It is also helpful if you thought you were over an emotional problem and it keeps coming back. This pt. is also good for stiff necks.)

GV-15 Mute's Gate (sea of bone marrow and a good pt. for muteness)

GV-16 Wind Mansion (Window of the Sky, sea of bone marrow)

GV-17 Brain Door (use acupressure only)

GV-18 Strength Divider

GV-19 Posterior Summit (sea of bone marrow)

GV-20 Meeting of 1000 Ancestors (sea of bone marrow, External Dragon pt. and good pt. for epilepsy and to calm the spirit)

GV-21 Anterior Summit

GV-22 Skull Meeting

GV-23 Upper Star

GV-24 Spirit Hall

GV-24.5 This pt. has no name but it is approximately in the location of the third eye.

GV-25 White Bone Hole

GV-26 Middle of Man

GV-27 Correct Exchange

GV-28 Mouth Crossing (I recommend using acupressure only.)

121

CHAPTER 23

SPECIAL POINTS

The following points are considered special points that have been used for common ailments over the years. You may want to explore these along with the other points you are using. These points were gleaned from a variety of sources.

These may be used as points to treat chronic conditions or first aid points for acute conditions. Remember, if you sting the extremities (arms and legs) within the first 2 - 3months of treatment you may have a great deal of swelling. I recommend that if you want to use these points, you do so in conjunction with the five element points.

ALLERGIES: LV-3, CO-4 & 11, TH-5, BL-10, K-27, CV-6, ST-36

ANEMIA: BL-38

ANKLE PROBLEMS: K-3 & 6, BL-60 & 62, GB-40

ASTHMA: GV-10, HP-8, L-10

ANXIETY: BL-10, TH-15, CV-17, HP-3 & 6, H-7

ARM PROBLEMS: TH-9,14, & 15, GB-20 & 21

ARTHRITIS: CO-4 & 11, TH-5 & 6, ST-36 & 39, GB-20
    OF THE KNEE: BL-54 & 55

BACK PAIN: BL-23, 25, 47, 48, 50, 51 & 54, CV-6, SP-8

BALANCE: TH-3

BELL'S PALSY: SI-5

BLADDER PROBLEMS: BL-58 & 65, LV-8 , K-2, Sting in pubic hair.

BLURRED VISION: BL-66, K-4, LV-3

BONE MARROW PROBLEMS: GB-39

COLDS/FLU: GB-20, K-27, CO-4, BL-10, CV-22

COLD LIMBS: ST-37, SP-2

CONSTIPATION: CV-6, ST-36, CO-4 & 11, BL-25 & 28

CO-ORDINATION PROBLEMS: TH-8, GB-34, 37 & 40

CORTISONE PRODUCTION: GB-39

COUGHS: ST-43, L-7 & 9

CHRONIC FATIGUE: L-1, GB-20 & 21, TH-2, 3, 5, 14, & 15, HP-6, ST-36, BL-23 & 47, CV-6, LV-3, SP-5 & 6, CO-15 & 16, SI-10, & SI-12 - 14

CRAMPS, SPASMS: BL-52, 53, 56 & 57, LV-3 & 4, K-9, GB-34 & GB-37

DEPRESSION : TH-5, CV-17, L-1, K-27, BL-1O, 23, 38 & 47, GV-19, 20 & 21, GB-20, CO-7, HP-6, ST-9 & 10

DEPRESSION BEFORE PERIOD: K-4

DIARRHEA: ST-36, LV-2, CV-6, SP-4

DIZZINESS: TH-3

EAR PROBLEMS: K-3, TH-2

ELBOW PROBLEMS: L-6, CO-11

EPILEPSY: GV-9, HP-9, ST-36 & 41, SI-3, TH-8

123

EYE PROBLEMS: GV-14, GB-1 (with care), 37 & 20, CO-4
    BLURRED VISION: BL-66, LV-3, K-4

FINGER PROBLEMS: TH-4, L-9

FRUSTRATION: GB-20, 21 & 30, BL-48, L-1, CV-17, CV -12

GOITER: GB-38, CO-10

GOUT: ST-41

HANDS (HARD TO GRASP THINGS): TH-4, L-9 , SI-9

HAIR (FALLING OUT): ST-39

HIP: GB-28, 29 & 30
    IF YOU HAVE A HIP PROBLEM ON ONE SIDE DO CO-18 ON
    THE OTHER SIDE OF THE BODY

HEADACHES: GB-20 & 41, BL-10, CO-4, LV-3
    FOR HEADACHES AT THE TOP OF THE HEAD: BL-6 & 7

HOT FLASHES: K-1 & 2, GB-2, CO-4, K-27, CV-17, GV-20

IMMUNE SYSTEM: K-3 & 27, CV-6 & 17, ST-36, LV-3, BL-23,
    BL 36 - 40, & 47, CO -11, TH-5 & 14, SI-14

INSOMNIA: SP-6, GB-2, BL-10, 38, 61 & 62, H-7, HP-6, CV-17,
    K-6 & 25, L-9

KNEE PROBLEMS: CO-9, ST-35 & 36, GB-34 & 44, LV-7 & 8,
    K-10, SP-9, BL-53, 54 & 61

MEMORY/CONCENTRATION: GV-20, GB-20, BL-10, CV-17,
    ST-36, LV-3

MIGRAINES: K-3, LV-3

NECK PAIN: GV-16, GB-20 & 21, TH-15 & 16, BL-6, 12 & 20

NECK, STIFF: SI-3, 16 & 17, BL-10, 54, 60, 64, 66, ST-6, GV-19

NIGHT SWEATS: BL -54, K-2

NUMBNESS (GENERAL): SP-6 & 9, TH-1
    HANDS & ARMS: L-11
    LEGS: CO-9

PAIN (UPPER BODY): GB-20, CO-4

PAIN (LOWER BODY): ST-36, K-3, GB-20, BL-60

PARALYSIS: GB-37, ST-40, GV-2

PMS/CRAMPS: SP-4, 6, 12 & 13, BL-27 through 34 & 48, CV-4 & 6

RHEUMATISM (NECK & SHOULDERS): BL-8, GB-41

RIGIDITY: CO-2, GV-5 & 12

SCIATICA: BL-10, 23, 47, 48, 50, 54, 60, 65, CV-6, GB-20, 30 & 40

SKIN DISORDERS: BL-10, 23 & 47, ST-36 & 44, L-10

SHOULDER, FROZEN: TH-1 & 4, CO-1 & 2, GV-13, & also treat
    BL-62 on the opposite side of the shoulder problem.

SHOULDER PAIN: GB-20 & 21, TH-14, 15 & 16, L-6, CO-15 &16,
    BL-36, SI-10 - 14

SPASMS: LV-6, GB-34 & 37, LV-3

SPEECH: GB-44, CO-8, ST-40

SPINE PROBLEMS: BL-62, K-5, GV-1 - 15

TINNITUS: BL-63, CO-5, ST-36, SI-2, 4, & 5

125

VERTIGO: SI-7

WEAKNESS: BL-58, K-9, LV-6, ST-38

WRIST-PAIN: TH-4,TH-5,HP-7,HP-6

CHAPTER 24

MAJOR BLOCKS

If you feel "stuck" or that you've hit a plateau, you may have a major block. It may be time to consider correcting this block. A major block is like a garden hose that is all twisted or has knots in it. You may have to unravel these knots to have a breakthrough.

There are several major blocks you can look into. It is best if they can be corrected by acupuncture needles. If your insurance does not cover acupuncture, you cannot afford it on your own, or if there is no acupuncturist in your area, you can consider stinging yourself on the recommended acupuncture points.

These treatments should be used after the swelling and itching reactions subside—this is usually after the first month or so. These treatments assist the healing process by either cleansing stagnant energy or by correcting chronic blockages in the flow of Ch'i. In most of these treatments, you sting all of the indicated points in one session. Generally, you may want to limit your treatments to one of these blocks at a time. The points listed as Windows and Entry/Exit blocks can be done as needed; you may want to add one or two of these points as part of a treatment plan derived from the five element work.

THE INTERNAL DRAGONS

This treatment is needed for one who feels stuck in an emotion: anger, joy, worry, grief, or anxiety (fear). It is called the Internal Dragons because it feels like something is coming at you from the inside. This is predominantly an emotional treatment and is therefore very good for depression. Dragons bring good luck in Oriental medicine.

This condition may come from a trauma or an ongoing emotional situation. Here are four indications to signal whether the Internal Dragons are present (usually all indications are present but not always):

127

1.   The person may feel possessed on the inside by something outside of himself, in this case an illness.

2.   The patient has trouble making eye contact. He doesn't look you in the eye. You may have the feeling that he is avoiding looking at you in general. You will feel like you are having trouble connecting with this person. He seems distant and far away. It may feel like "nobody's home."

3.   The person's life may seem very chaotic.

4.   His symptoms have been persistent over a long period of time. Statements that go with the Internal Dragons may sound similar to these:

"I have a rip in my soul that I just can't get around."
"This isn't me. I feel like something else has taken over."
"I'm feeling out of control; I feel like the rage (worry, grief) has taken over and is controlling me."

To release the 7 Internal Dragons you need the following points:

The master point below CV-15
Stomach-25 (bilaterally)
Stomach-32 (bilaterally)
Stomach-41(bilaterally)

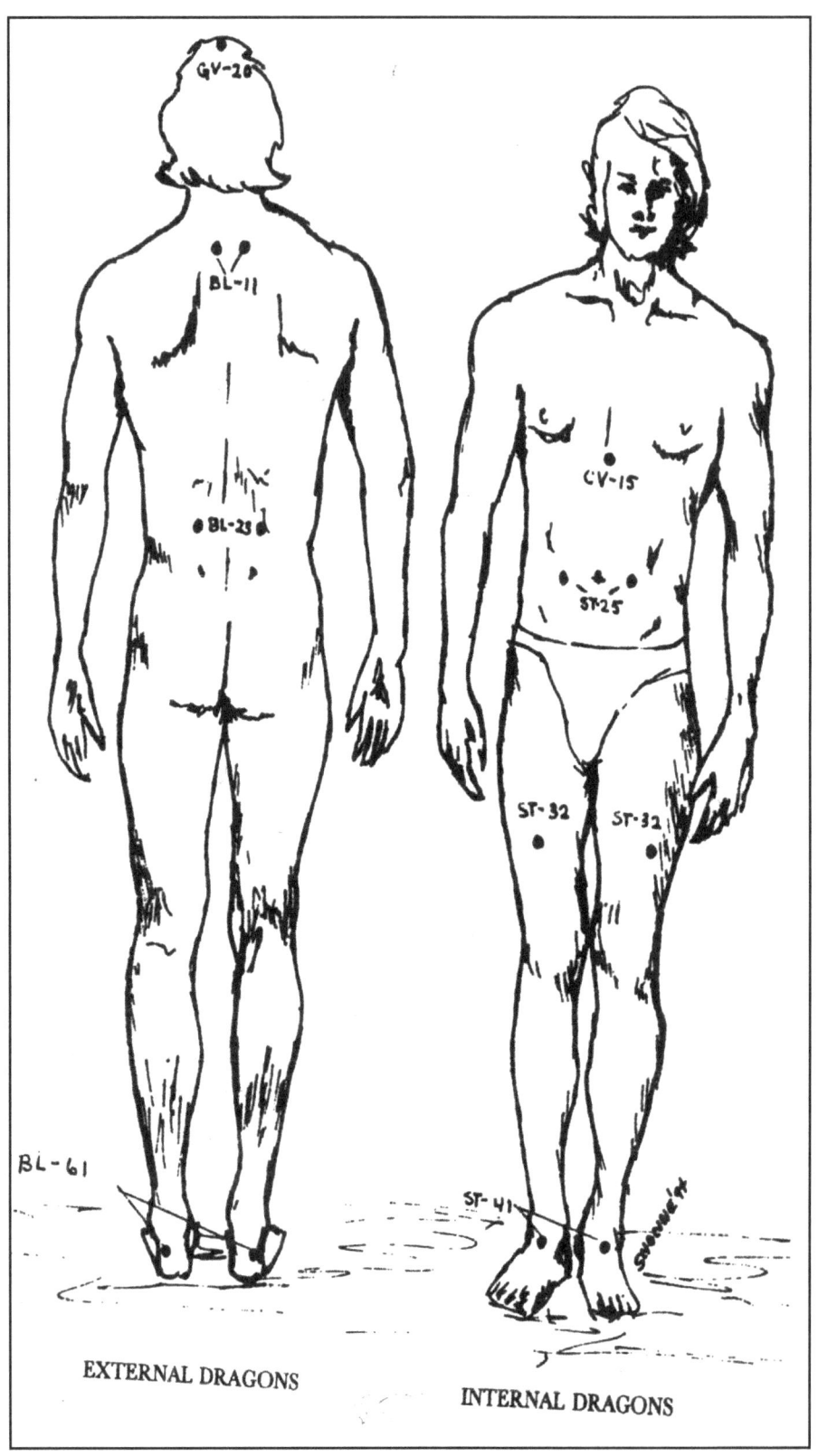

THE EXTERNAL DRAGONS

This treatment is needed if something came at you from the outside. It could be a disease, a car accident, a rape, a fall, or a major trauma of some kind. This condition may also be present if you were exposed to "the elements" for a period of time, for example: dampness, humidity, fire, heat, cold, wind, or dryness.

Let's say you were outside on a very cold day and ever since then you have not been able to get warm. An extreme example of that would be frostbite. Another example might be if your house caught on fire and you just barely escaped. In this case, you would be exposed to the external fire and heat and perhaps even wind. This would be a perfect example of how the Internal and External Dragons might be needed. If you narrowly escaped from a fire, there would probably be a lot of fear associated with that experience. Then you would treat both the Internal and External Dragons.

The same four indications may be present as listed above for the Internal Dragons, with the main difference being that the person feels very strongly that something came at them from the outside.

Here are the points needed to release the 7 External Dragons and correct the situation:

GV-20
Bladder 11 (bilaterally)
Bladder 23 (bilaterally)
Bladder 61 (bilaterally)

If the person regains good eye contact, then you know the pattern has been broken. I wish you good luck. It is harder to get results if this condition persists. Please keep me posted on your results.

AGGRESSIVE ENERGY (AE)-CLEAR JAKI

If left uncontrolled long enough, the K'o cycle will become self-destructive. We call this condition "aggressive energy." When this situation arises, the patient is likely to show some self-destructive behaviors (like drug abuse, car accidents, suicide attempts, etc.) She may also be prone to have illnesses where the body attacks itself, such as cancer, MS, lupus, and diseases which are thought to be auto-immune in nature. Aggressive Energy can be drained fairly easily with acupuncture needles.

Aggressive Energy is an invasive energy that knocks us off balance. It is harmful energy that is aimed at controlling the grandson instead of feeding the son. Looking at the chart of the five elements, you can note that the K'o cycle reaches across along the path of the star, rather than around the circle, which is the path of the Shen cycle. It is energy that stagnates and then aggressively moves across the K'o cycle; a metaphor for this would be that the grandmother is sick and turns on the grandchild. AE is a step beyond reasonable control. It is very destructive and deep seated. The danger is to the yin organs: the liver, the heart, the heart protector, the spleen, the lungs, and the kidneys. AE can be triggered by an acute or devastating trauma or a chronic condition, i.e., pain or illness.

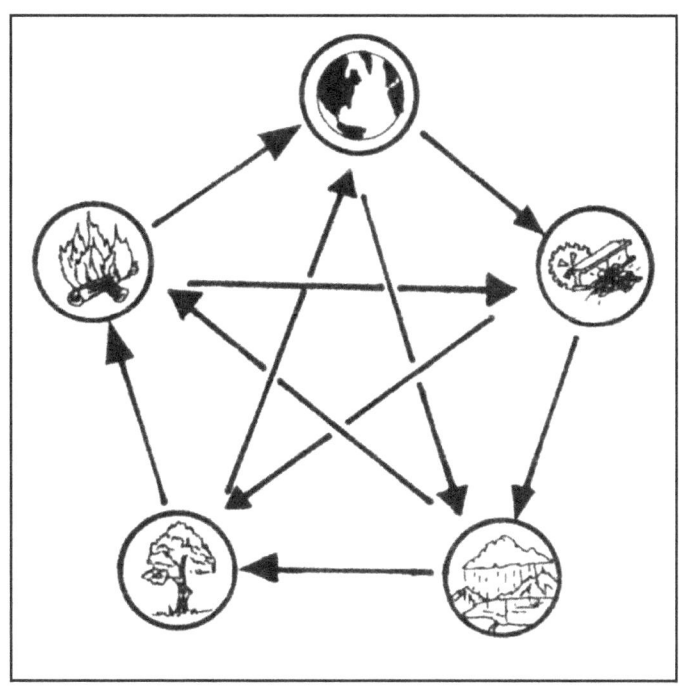

K'o Cycle: Aggressive energy moves across the K'o cycle, which occurs when the grandmother is out of balance and the cycle of control becomes destructive

So if you have symptoms in a pair of elements which are connected as grandmother—grandchild, then you may have Aggressive Energy. For example, if you have trouble in the wood element (e.g., menstrual cramps, problems with tendons and ligaments, one-sided headaches, trouble making decisions) and you also have symptoms in the earth element (e.g., craving sweets, stomach or digestion issues, food allergies, leg and feet problems, feeling misunderstood) then you may have Aggressive Energy.

Another indication that you may have Aggressive Energy is having a chronic illness, especially one thought to be an auto-immune disease, like cancer, MS, lupus, AIDS, etc.

A third indication for Aggressive Energy is that you've had a major trauma.

If you have Aggressive Energy you are hard to be around. You are really struggling. You may also be self-absorbed or have some self-destructive behaviors: car accidents, addictions, destructive relationships that you stay stuck in, to name a few.

Also, if you are feeling blocked in your response to Bee Venom Therapy, then you may want to try the Aggressive Energy treatment.

OK, so now you think you have Aggressive Energy . . . what do you do now? An acupuncturist can drain this for you. You may want to consider this; it is a very simple procedure. Basically, 12 needles are inserted (very superficially) in the back Shu points for the yin organs. (Three test needles are also used for placebos, or control needles in non-points.) Here is a list of the points that are used. All points are done bilaterally:

BLADDER-13 (FOR THE LUNGS)
BLADDER-14 (FOR THE HEART PROTECTOR)
BLADDER-15 (FOR THE HEART)
BLADDER-18 (FOR THE LIVER)
BLADDER-20 (FOR THE SPLEEN)
BLADDER-23 (FOR THE KIDNEYS)

The acupuncturist should put the needles in very superficially, with no manipulation. If you have AE, a redness will develop around the needle. Sometimes there will be no redness but the person will still benefit from the treatment. What the acupuncturist is doing is draining the harmful energy out of the organs where it has gotten stuck. I like to look at it this way: think of a teapot that is on the stove. The burner is on and the water in the teapot is now boiling. But unfortunately, the hole in the teapot is plugged up and there is no place for the steam to escape. What we are doing, by draining the AE, is making a hole is the teapot for the steam to escape so it doesn't stay so bottled up.

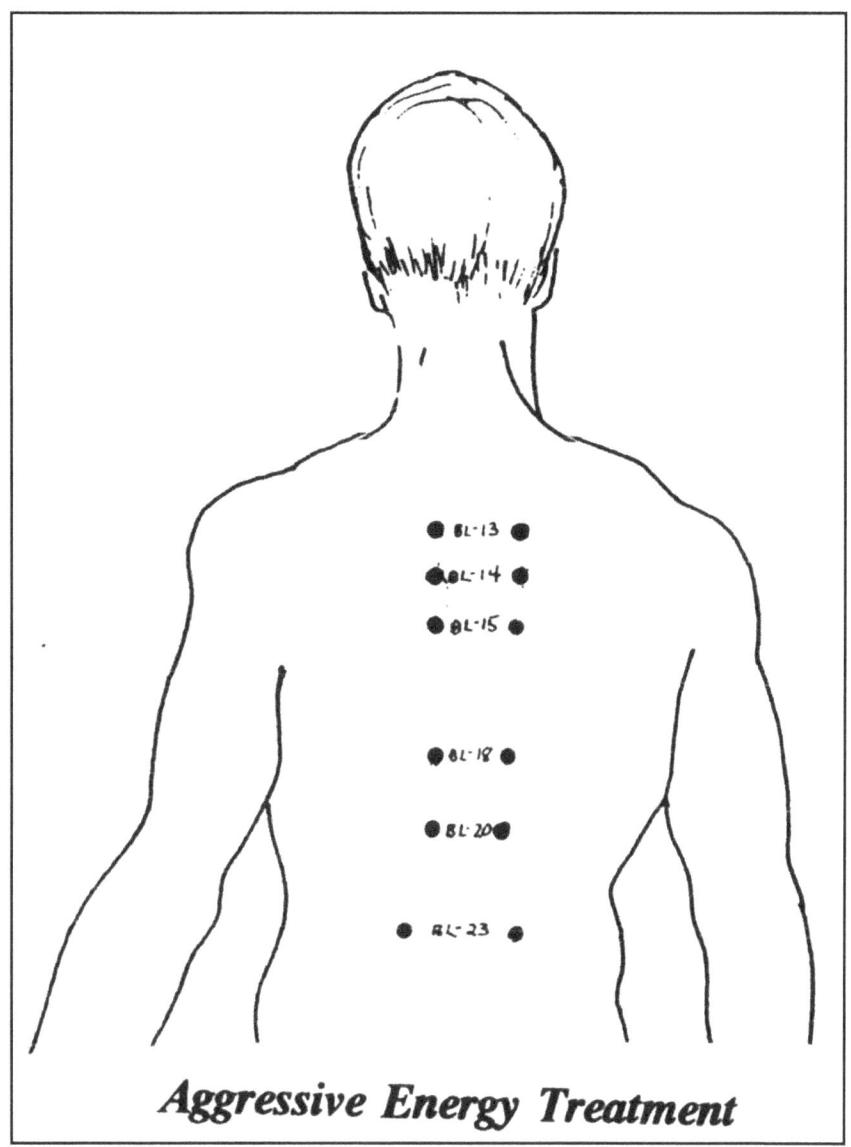

Aggressive Energy Treatment

What about those of you who are unable to find or go to an acupuncturist? If you think you may have Aggressive Energy, my suggestion to you is to have someone sting you on the points illustrated above. It may not be quite as good as an acupuncture treatment, but it's definitely a step in the right direction.

A HUSBAND - WIFE IMBALANCE (H - W)

In general, you will not know if you need this treatment without a trained acupuncturist to assess your pulses, but is worth mentioning because it is a major stumbling block to your health if you have it. The pulses on the left hand are considered to be the Husband and the right hand is the Wife. The Law of Husband and Wife states that the pulses

134

on the left hand (Husband) should be slightly stronger qualitatively and quantitatively than the right hand pulses (the Wife). If this is reversed, it is called a Husband-Wife Imbalance. This is serious and must be corrected immediately. There is a sense of chaos with this condition. The person may feel like they are being torn apart or that they have to give up a part of themselves to survive. The indications for a Husband - Wife Imbalance are:

Pulse Picture - This is the main indication. The pulses on the left hand (the Husband) are supposed to be stronger qualitatively and quantitatively than the pulses on the right hand (the Wife). In a H - W this would be reversed; the pulses on the right hand will be stronger than the pulses on the left.

A Bad Marriage/relationship - If it is badly out of balance, they may feel like they have to give up a part of themselves to survive.

Job - They have a very demanding job and they don't get much out of it. They may say, "This job is killing me!"

Health - They may be chronically ill and there is chaos to their energy.

They may feel split and are trying to bring themselves into balance.

Here are the points an acupuncturist would tonify to correct this condition:

KIDNEY-7 (is not on chart)
BLADDER-67
KIDNEY-3
BLADDER-64
LIVER-3
GALL BLADDER-40
LIVER-4

If the H - W is not broken after doing these points, the practitioner can tonify the following points:

BLADDER-15
BLADDER-23
BLADDER-18
BLADDER- 27
BLADDER-19
BLADDER-28

If the H - W is still not broken, then the acupuncturist can sedate the following points: These points should not be stung because bee stings will stimulate or tonify the points rather than sedate them. These points can be massaged with a counter-clockwise motion instead.

LUNG-5
COLON-2
STOMACH-42
SPLEEN-3
HEART PROTECTOR-7
THREE HEATER-4

When the H - W is finally broken, stinging the following two points will keep the imbalance from coming back:

HEART-7
SMALL INTESTINE-4

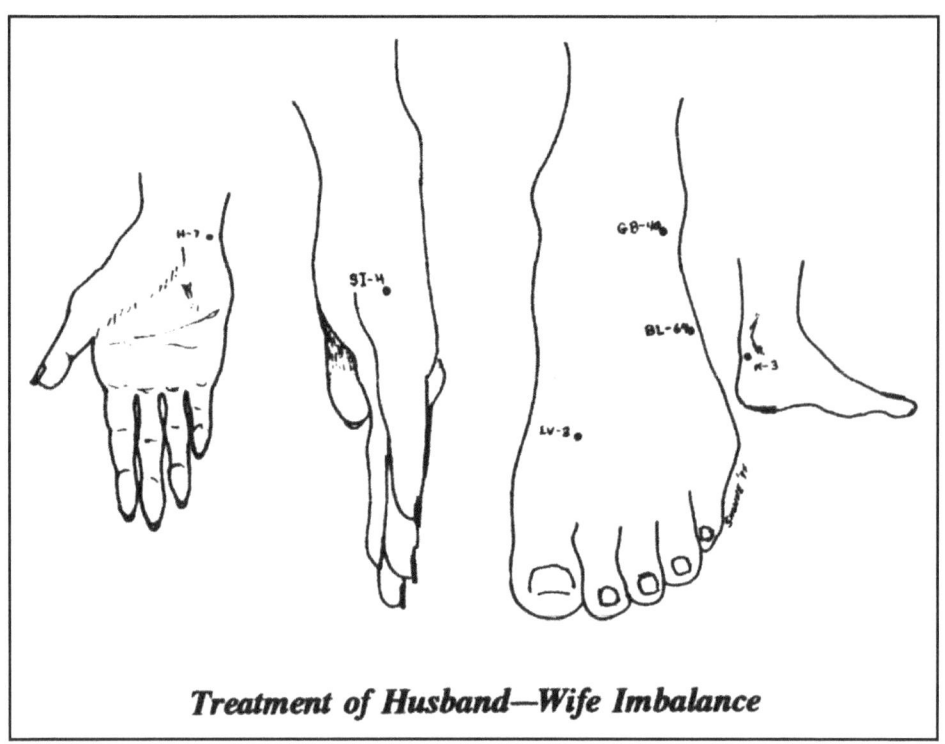

Treatment of Husband—Wife Imbalance

Treatment of Husband - Wife Imbalance

The Chinese pulse picture is very different than the Western pulse picture. As an acupuncturist I am looking at the quantity and quality of the pulse, but I am not counting the number of beats per minute. There are twelve positions (6 on each wrist) to check the pulse for each of the 12 meridians. The goal is to have all pulses in balance and harmony.

Good luck trying to break this major block. I have done it successfully with bees alone and no needles. Just remember that if you do all the points on the feet within the 3 months or so you will get a great deal of swelling. I would therefore save this treatment until the fourth month, after you have crept down the leg, calf, ankle, and foot with test stings.

WINDOWS OF THE SKY

There are 11 Windows of the Sky. Most of them are on the neck or close to it. A Window is indicated when the person really wants a breakthrough. They have to be ready. They will ask you for it, and even beg for it.

They may say, "I really want to see what happened in my childhood." Or they may say, "I'm at the end of my rope; I have to break through all this soon!" They may also state that they "feel cut off from the neck down."

In general, when we go through a major trauma in childhood, we shut down. In this case, we close down our Windows. Tonifying a Window will help the person to open up more. Windows bring the body, mind, and spirit together. You can open up a Window with the bees, because they will tonify the point. If you want to sedate a Window when it's too open, you would probably need to use a needle or use acupressure on the point (the acupuncturist would turn it counter-clockwise). In general I don't recommend trying to sedate a point with bee stings, because (as I stated earlier) the very act of stinging the person will stimulate rather than sedate the point.

The following points are Windows of the Sky:

SMALL INTESTINE-16
SMALL INTESTINE-17
BLADDER -10
HEART PROTECTOR-1 (MEN)(Forbidden in WOMEN)
HEART PROTECTOR -2 (WOMEN)
THREE HEATER-16
LUNG-3
COLON -18
STOMACH-9
CONCEPTION VESSEL-22
GOVERNOR VESSEL-16

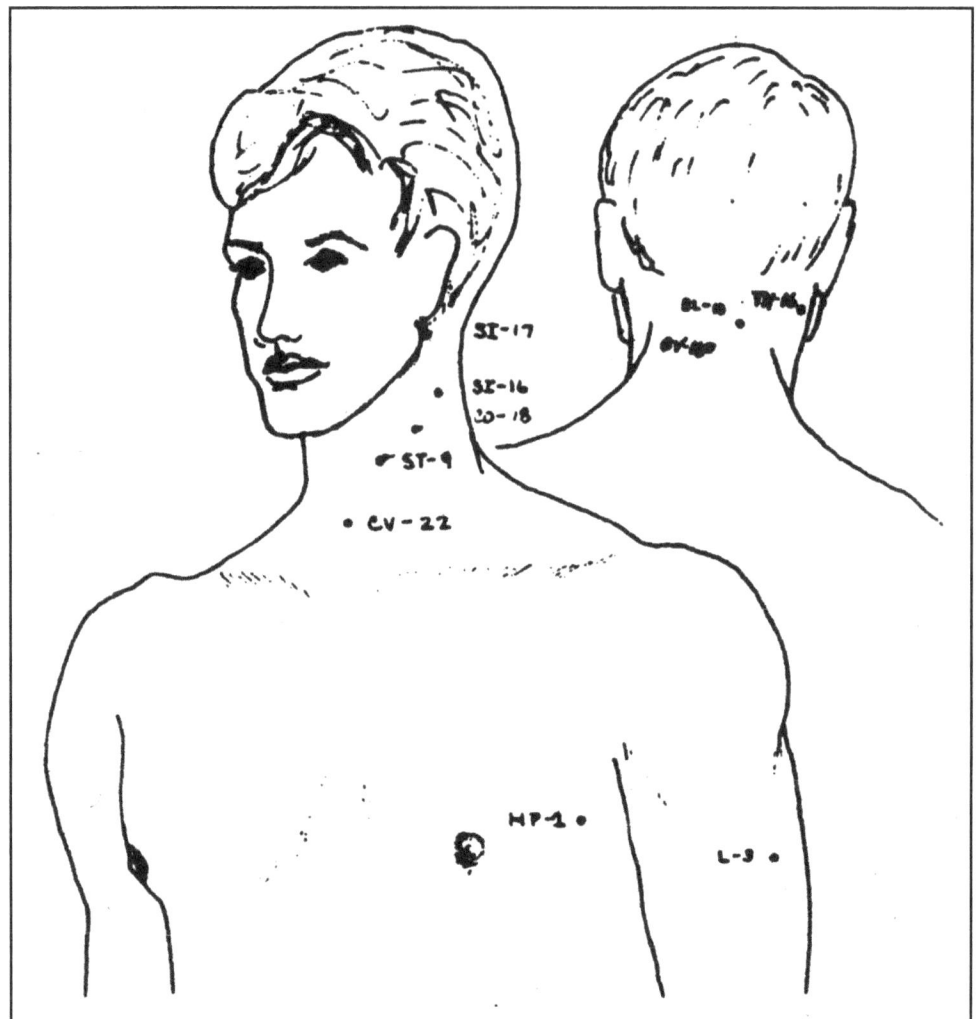

ENTRY/EXIT BLOCKS

Each pathway has an entry and an exit point. These points are located at or near the beginning and end of each pathway, and are the points from which the energy flows from one meridian to the next. This energy flows in the same order described in the Chinese Clock. The direction of flow in the Chinese Clock is based on the anatomical relationship between the meridians. The heart pathway, for example, flows from H-1 down the arm to the inside of the little finger, which is the exit point, H-9. The very first point on the small intestine, SI-1, is on the outside of the little finger. The Ch'i flows across the nail from H-9 to SI-1, the small intestine entry point. The Chinese Clock thus shows the energy flowing from the heart to the small intestine.

139

The entry/exit points are like gateways, and can be rusted shut or open. This would be an entry/exit block. It can be easily corrected by treating the entry and exit points on one pathway and perhaps the entry and exit points on the following pathway. By "following pathway," I mean the next pathway according to the Chinese Clock. There are 12 major pathways through which energy flows in the body. There are 24 hours in a day; therefore each pathway is at its peak for two hours every day. If you are having symptoms at the same time every day, you probably have an entry/exit block. You will need to flush out the pathway.

For example, the time of day that goes with the liver pathway is 1 a.m. to 3 a.m. ("sun" time, not daylight savings time). If you are consistently waking up in the middle of the night at this time, it means you have an entry/exit block on the liver. You would need to treat LV-1 and LV-13 and 14 (the liver has two exit points, which is unusual). But if you are waking up at 3:15 a.m. that is in the lung time, so in this case you might want to treat the liver exit points and the entry point on the lungs, L-1. Or here's another very classic pattern: a person who has had a death in the family may wake up at 3 a.m. (the lung time, a time of grief and letting go, feelings of loss). If there is also anger involved, you may wake up at 2 or 2:30 a.m. and not be able to get back to sleep. This is the transition time between anger and grief. This condition indicates an entry/exit block between the liver and the lungs.

What this means is that the energy around the Chinese Clock is not functioning properly. If there is a block on this level, the energy is unable to flow smoothly in its normal path from the exit point of one meridian to the entry point of the next meridian. So a bottleneck, blockage, or excess starts to build up at the exit point. Think of a garden hose with kinks or knots in it. The water cannot flow through it very well and so not much water will come out when you try to water your plants.

This condition can be very frustrating, because no matter what the person does, they can't seem to break the pattern. The condition persists, sometimes for years. Medications to treat the symptoms only cover up the problem like a band-aid. An acupuncturist can correct this block in just a matter of minutes. Now you can see why we ask people what their favorite time of day is and what their worst time of day is. An entry/exit block can be detected on the pulses.

You probably need to use entry/exit points when two or more consecutive pathways are having trouble. In this case, consecutive means according to the Chinese Clock. This means that you would have symptoms at the same time almost every day. You may also need to use entry/exit points when the patient is doing well and then all of a sudden the old symptoms come back.

entry	exit
GB-1 take care	GB-41
LV-1	LV-14 (LV -13)
H-1	H-9
SI-1	SI-19
HP-1 (MEN)	HP-8
HP-2 (WOMEN)	HP-8
TH-1	TH-22
ST-1	ST-42
SP-1	SP-21
L-1	L-7
CO-4	CO-20 (take care)
BL-1	BL-67
K-1	K-22
CV-1 (take care)	CV-24 (take care)
GV-1	GV-28 (take care)

SCARS

Because scars block the flow of energy in the body, they are also considered major blocks. These should be treated by stinging directly on the scar and to either side of the scar. This will promote healing by bringing blood to the area. Also, you can sting the closest acupuncture points above and below the scar. If a scar cuts through a pathway, energy may be blocked.

Good luck, may the dragons be with you as you wing your way.

CHAPTER 25

CONCLUSION

"Your Life is Your Message"

The Soul has a curriculum to transcend life's lessons. It also has a destiny to fulfill. Classical and Bee - Acupuncture awaken the spirit in each of us to do what we came here to do. We each have a mission to complete. Everyone who lived did not live in vain. Each of us has a reason and a purpose to be here.

The fundamental question you will ask is: Why is this happening to me? And the answer is: Do you want to be healed? Once you say yes, then healing can take place. If you are "unable" to or "incapable of saying yes, then you are still living in the past. Healing takes place in the moment. The past is only important after the present has been explored.

The moment is your life. And as Mahatma Gandhi said, "Your life is your message." Healing takes place spirit to spirit. If I don't know who you are, I can serve you. If I know who you are, I am you. And that makes all the difference. We must bring the healing out of the treatment and into your life. There is no beginning and there is no end. We must weave the moment together like "The Web that has no Weaver" (T.Kaptchuk).

Healing takes place in the presence of a cultivated being; you are a pioneer in a whole new field of medicine. Along with the bees, you are healing yourself. Through your presence and vibration transformation occurs. The gift of the venom is to serve as a catalyst, midwife, alchemist, and guide for that transformation. The Pearl of Great Price is to alleviate suffering. Honor the relevance of your feelings and symptoms. Find meaning in your suffering. Healing is not the absence of symptoms. People are healed, not "cured." Develop an emotional bond and befriend your symptoms. Trust the healing process, not the end result. Healing is a continuous way of living. Explore the depth of your present feelings. Remember that everything we experience as suffering can become healing.

Before you get ready to sting yourself or others, you need to focus and become an empty vessel. Every time you sting yourself, it is for the first time. Maintain your humility. Come from a place of stability and groundedness. See yourself as if you were already whole. Remember: you are somebody's mother, father, sister, brother, grandmother, etc. Be open. Be innocent. Suspend thinking, judgment, expectations, and "right" decisions. Bring back states of innocence and new beginnings. Give yourself hope (Liver 14 - Gate of Hope). Start a new chapter in your life (Liver 13 - Chapter Gate).

Most of all BE PRESENT. This is the crucial factor. Take time to listen to yourself. Your focus and intention needs to be bringing the body, mind, and spirit together. Your bee sting is a conduit of intentionality. Release fear and let it go, if you can. Be honest with your feelings. Your body language illuminates the path you must follow. Take on the challenge of being present with your suffering.

Don't get caught up in the past. Fear is energized by worrying. You can't be whole if you are stuck in the past. Fear can also be anticipation of something in the future. Help yourself feel whole in the present moment. "What would you be feeling right now, if you weren't worried?" Break away from rigidity.

Healing is a willingness to heal thyself. It is a living state of awareness and empowerment. Become more responsible for your life. See the beauty in the moment. Create your own reality, your own salvation. If you could write the script, what would you do with the rest of your life? If you only had 9 months to live…what would you do with your time? Be responsible to the reality of now. If you can find a way to embrace your suffering you won't be afraid of it.

We must examine the "stuckness" where we are all trapped. We must bring our whole being to stinging each acupuncture point. We help to open or close the doors or portals of perception. Trust is needed to develop this kind of intimacy. We need to focus on validating our strengths.

We need to be able to die at any moment. But it is more important to decide how to live. Everything has the possibility of turning into its opposite. The Starpoint within us will guide our way home. If I could wave a magic wand, I would wish for you to find grace in your world, peace in your life, and that you come to inherit your wisdom and your destiny.